A Child is Waiting

Vernon L. James, MD
Emeritus Fellow, American Academy of Pediatrics

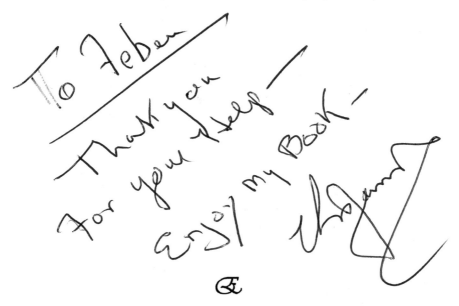

Strategic Book Publishing and Rights Co.

Copyright © 2016 Vernon James. All rights reserved.

No part of this book may be reproduced or transmitted in any form or by any means, graphic, electronic, or mechanical, including photocopying, recording, taping, or by any information storage retrieval system, without the permission, in writing, of the publisher. For more information, send an email to support@sbpra.net, Attention Subsidiary Rights Department.

Strategic Book Publishing and Rights Co., LLC
USA I Singapore

For information about special discounts for bulk purchases, please contact Strategic Book Publishing and Rights Co. Special Sales, at bookorder@sbpra.net.

ISBN: 978-1-68181-424-7

Book Design: Suzanne Kelly

Also by the author
A Community of Healers

Acknowledgements

My deep-felt gratitude goes to all of those wonderful families and children who chose me as their Pediatrician.

A special thank you goes to those families who have allowed me to share their stories and photos in this book.

Bill Allew, photographer, who made it possible to include the photos and illustrations.

An expression of gratitude is due to my brother, Frank James, MD who read the manuscript and offered excellent suggestions. More importantly, he provided me with continual support and guidance.

I especially want to thank my wife, my partner, Dr. Dessie James, for her unwavering support and encouragement.

Table of Contents

Introduction ix

Chapter One   Polio 1

Chapter Two   Contagious Diseases 7
                     Diphtheria, Mumps, Rubella

Chapter Three   Contagious Diseases 13
                     Pertussis, Measles

Chapter Four   Prematurity 18

Chapter Five   Newborn Screening 23

Chapter Six   Chromosomes 30
                     Down Syndrome

Chapter Seven   Genes 38
                     Fragile X, Angelman Syndrome,
                     Prader-Willi Syndrome

Chapter Eight   Congenital Defects 44
                     Spina Bifida, Hydrocephalus

Chapter Nine   Genetic Defect 50
                     Cystic Fibrosis

Chapter Ten   Prenatal Attacks 56
                     AIDs, CMV, Rh Factor

Chapter Eleven   Cerebral Palsy 63

Chapter Twelve   Muscular Dystrophy 67

Chapter Thirteen Deaf and Hard of Hearing 72

Chapter Fourteen Intellectual Developmental
                     Disability 80

Chapter Fifteen	Autism	86
Chapter Sixteen	Diabetes	93
Chapter Seventeen	Overweight and Obesity	99
Chapter Eighteen	Visual Impairment and Blindness	104
Chapter Nineteen	Problems of Attention, Learning Differences	110
Chapter Twenty	Abuse and Neglect	116
Chapter Twenty-One	Cancer	122
Chapter Twenty-Two	Ethical Issues	127
Chapter Twenty-Three	Parent Power	137
Chapter Twenty-Four	Death	145
Epilogue		149
Index		151

Introduction

When the DNA from a father and a mother come together, a new and miraculous organism is conceived. About seven weeks after conception, this fetus begins random movements, which become purposeful movements as it matures. By the fifteenth week, taste buds are formed. Olfactory (smell) cells begin to function around twenty-fourth week. A fetus begins to hear between twenty-four and twenty-seven weeks. Vision takes the longest, with the eyes opening at twenty-eight weeks, although we are not sure what they can see.

In spite of all this maturity, newborns come into this world as totally helpless creatures. As human newborns, we are the most helpless of all creatures and are completely dependent on those around us for life, sustenance, and survival. We remain dependent until we mature and are able to provide for own needs.

Humans are vulnerable to attacks from the moment of conception and throughout life. We are vulnerable to the effects of flawed chromosomes and genes, to attacks by multiple diseases, to attacks by those who should protect us, to the environment in which we live, and even to laws passed by governments about which we have no say. Children can't even vote for those who make the laws governing their lives. They have no vote on the family we are born into, where we live, how we are taught, how we are treated, or even what's for supper. They depend on a vast number of adults for their well-being.

Childhood is not a democratic process.

Children have rights, and they are simple: the right to happiness and joy, to safety and protection, to good health and effective treatment and to the opportunity to reach their highest potential.

Vernon L. James, MD

To protect these rights requires the advocacy of every entity in the child's community. This obviously includes the child's parents and extended family, but it also includes neighbors and friends, physicians and therapists, schools and teachers, coaches, governments, and all of society.

To be an active advocate for children is the highest calling any human being can undertake. It has taken me into many arenas of the world, exposed me to immeasurable experiences, and taught me that to be an advocate for children is to really live.

I have written this book:

- To present information in a different voice, to those who care for our vulnerable children
- To add to the knowledge of anyone who has a special needs child in their life
- To explain how a condition, disease, or handicap happens and how it interferes with children achieving their rights
- To help everyone realize that knowledge is power, hope is essential, and love is unqualified

In this book, I will describe many attacks on children, taken from my experience; some from the past, some attackers have been conquered, and some are viciously attacking children today. Each anecdote is taken from my life experiences in over fifty years of pediatrics. Each anecdote is a true experience, with the facts as I remember them today. Hopefully, each experience described will increase your knowledge, awareness, and insight on the condition described, and you will enjoy sharing the moment with me.

My prayer is that, as you read, you will realize how you may become an active advocate for children, wherever and whenever the opportunity gives you a call.

A child somewhere is waiting for you; maybe one of yours.

CHAPTER ONE

Polio

The basement room in the hospital was large, almost like a gymnasium. It was hard to look out the windows because they were small and at the top half of the room, but the flashes of lightning lit up the windows like fireflies. While sitting quietly at the desk, I watched the flashes as the storm moved closer. The desk was surrounded by thirteen iron lungs, each one holding a small child.

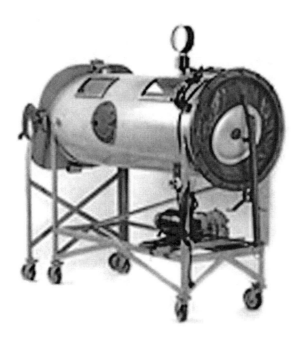

The silence of the room was broken by the mechanical whooshing as each lung brought life-preserving oxygen into the flail chest the child inside. Those children had the near-deadly experience of a tiny virus, the one that caused poliomyelitis, attacking their bodies. This cursed virus had ravaged their small bodies and paralyzed each child from the neck down. They could not move their arms or legs. It affected their diaphragms, so they could not breathe. The iron lungs breathed for them. It kept them alive. They were frightened and felt helplessly alone.

I was dead tired, having worked in the emergency room all day. Now I was on the midnight shift caring for these unfortunate children. Many children had been seen in the ER with polio. Fortunately, most of them had not developed the paralytic complication. The whole nation was in the midst of an epidemic. Just the year before, in 1954, there had been over 55,000 cases. Many of them had resulted in some form of paralysis.

Sitting in the semi-darkness, I remembered a special little girl I had seen in the ER earlier that night. She had a high fever, flushed face, and was covered with sweat. She said in a soft quiet voice that she was, "four years old" and her name was "Mindy." I could still see the black curls stuck to her forehead from the sweat that covered her brow, and could picture the frightened look in her eyes. Her spinal tap was positive for polio.

The paralysis gradually crept up her little body like a wave of cursed affliction. When it reached her chest, her breathing became labored. She needed an iron lung, but there were none available. We called all the other hospitals in the city, but their lungs were all full. We were devastated as her life slipped away. In my short medical career, this was my first encounter with death, with the finality of life. As a physician with years of study, a brain full of facts, quotes, and an overwhelming amount of information, I was not prepared or ready to face this finality. I had thought I could do everything, but the death of a child was beyond all this training. There was no choice. I had to try to help these children under my care that night.

Shaking off the wave of sadness, I rose from the desk to check each child in the lungs. Although life-saving, the experience of being placed in an iron lung is extremely frightening. Each lung is a large cylinder with portholes on each side so a caretaker can reach inside and change diapers, give a bath, change clothing, or do whatever else is needed. The child is placed in the cylinder with only the head outside on a pillow. A mirror is placed over the head so the child can see around the room.

Those eyes followed me as I quietly moved around their small world. They were completely helpless, as the disease had robbed them of the ability to use their arms, legs, and hands, and even to talk. A large bellows is at the end of the cylinder and moves the air into their lungs. It makes a loud "whooshing" noise as it moves in and out. My job was to regulate the rate and pressures of the bellows.

As the air moved out of the chest, a child could say a word or so. Moving from one lung to another, I tried to be upbeat with each child.

A young boy with red hair and freckles said, *whoosh* . . . "Would you" . . . *whoosh* . . . "please scratch"... *whoosh* ... "my nose?"

A four-year-old girl said, *whoosh* . . . "When" . . . *whoosh* . . . "is my" . . . *whoosh* . . . "mommy" . . . *whoosh* . . . "coming?"

And so it went from one child to another.

Glancing at the windows, it seemed the storm was getting stronger and closer. The flashes of lightning were more intense and I could hear the crashes of thunder.

My mind wandered to the newest report that stated the new polio vaccine was now in clinical trials. How fantastic that would be if this horrible disease could be conquered. There had been several epidemics throughout the world. In 1916, there was a severe epidemic in Brooklyn, NY. Over 70,000 cats were slaughtered because it was mistakenly thought that cats spread the disease.

In 1937, a new organization was formed called the National Foundation for Infantile Paralysis with the support of President Franklin Roosevelt. Roosevelt was himself a polio victim who was paralyzed from the waist down in the polio epidemic in 1921. He was thirty-nine years old at the time and never regained the use of his legs. The foundation raised millions of dollars through the March of Dimes. The foundation supported research, treatment, and rehabilitation of many polio victims. It was clear that a prevention was desperately needed. In 1935, a trial of live polio virus injections as a vaccine was a disaster, resulting in numerous cases of active polio.

> *"If you spent two years in bed, trying to wiggle your big toe,*
>
> *After that everything would seem easy"*
>
> *Franklin D. Roosevelt, Polio Victim*
>
> *32 U.S. President 1933-1945*

In 1943, the foundation sent a researcher named Albert Sabin to North Africa to study a polio outbreak. Dr. Sabin went on to develop a polio vaccine based on the use of live but attenuated (changed) polio viruses. His vaccine was first tried in 1957 and licensed in 1962. The first vaccine, however, was developed by Dr. Jonas Salk, based on the use of killed viruses.

A double blind study was conducted in 1954 with a million children participating. Those brave parents and children were being given this first, untested vaccine developed by Dr. Salk. The newspaper called them "Polio Pioneers." It was a success and the vaccine was licensed in 1955. The most remarkable thing about this miraculous story was the total support of the public in raising money for this research. It was called The March of Dimes, and children all over the country collected dimes to support Dr. Salk, Dr. Sabin, and others who were searching for a vaccine. At that time, there was minimal government financial aid for research. This outpouring of public support made the development of a vaccine possible.

As I watched the children in the lungs, I prayed that the vaccine would be released soon. Maybe, just maybe, I would be the last intern to watch the suffering of precious kids being placed in iron lungs.

Suddenly, there was a bright flash of lightning and a crash of thunder. It sounded as if it was in the room. The electricity went out. All lights went out and the lungs stopped.

I panicked. The maintenance engineer would have to go to the emergency generators and turn them on. They were not automatic. Frantically, I tried to pump the bellows of each lung by hand. It was an impossible task. My heart felt like it was bursting as each child slipped away. Slowly, their eyes closed as the spark of life left their frail bodies. I couldn't breathe; the pain in my chest was excruciating and the lump in the throat wouldn't go away. The tears flowed and I experienced overwhelming pain. I can feel the same painful feeling and tears fill my eyes as I write this story. It will never go away.

Help came too late. They all died. All I could say was, "I tried, but I couldn't save them."

The chief came and sent me home for the rest of the night, as if that would erase the look in the eyes of those children that was burned in my brain forever.

The vaccine worked and has been given to children all over the world. We are thankful to many organizations that have supported worldwide dissemination. Perhaps the most effective has been Rotary International. Through their efforts, only three countries in the world—Afghanistan, Pakistan and Nigeria—still have polio cases.

In those countries, the vaccine has been prohibited by radical, misguided extremists. Many Rotarians have traveled all over the world to deliver and actually administer the vaccine to children. Many parents have been brave enough to allow this vaccine to be given to their children.

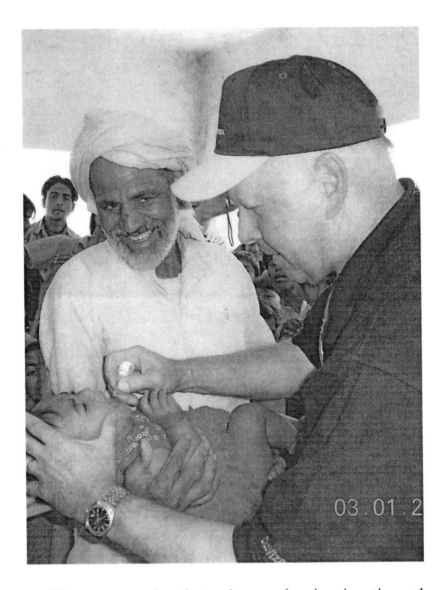

We must remember that as long as the virus is active and present anywhere in the world, there is the possibility of spread, and children anywhere could be attacked.

My prayer has almost been answered and, hopefully, no child will ever be put in an iron lung and no intern will ever have to care for a child paralyzed due to polio.

CHAPTER TWO

Contagious Diseases
Diphtheria, Mumps, Rubella

The emergency room was packed with people. Children were running around the room and probably spreading their germs. Unfortunately, some had been waiting just too long. The waiting room was painted a quiet color to calm people down, but it obviously wasn't working. There were rows and rows of chairs, all full. A few adults were standing and leaning against the wall.

I had just started back to work from the traumatic experience in the polio ward and other interns had promised they would see the polio-infected children. I was already tired from working on the wards all day. Standing in the doorway, I watched the chaos in the waiting room, realizing these children were here to see me. The head nurse said, "If you are the new intern, don't just stand there daydreaming. It's time to get to work. We're going to be here all night."

I slipped on my white coat, put the stethoscope around my neck, checked the new, Mont Blanc graduation gift pen in my pocket as the nurse handed me a chart. She said, "See this one next—he's pretty sick."

The chart was marked "contagious disease," so I put a mask across my nose. I hate wearing a mask. It seemed so impersonal and even seemed to scare the children. A three-year-old boy was having severe problems breathing. He had a high fever and his black hair was pasted across his forehead. His dark eyes were wide and full of fear. A large family of two older brothers, and a mother and father and a grandfather, crowded into the small room. They were all dressed in black and standing around the mother, who was holding the child. The men had beards and the women wore small white hats. I assumed they belonged to a religious group. The child was in a serious, life threatening condition.

The grandfather stood and took control. He was a tall thin gentleman with a thick black beard sprinkled with gray. He spoke in a clear, soft but firm voice. "Sir, this child is very ill and needs some of your medicine."

He was correct!

I noted there was something blocking the child's airway. His neck was swollen on both sides and he winced when it was touched. There was a thick greenish discharge coming from his nose. There was a bluish tint to his skin indicating a lack of oxygen in his blood. His pulse was very rapid and he breathed with difficulty getting his air in. I asked the child to open his mouth and was rewarded by a determined angry stare and shake of the head. The grandfather tried to get the child to open his mouth, but this little boy defiantly shook his head more vigorously. When it appeared that force was the next step, the child began to fight.

I remembered a story written by William Carlos Williams. It was called "The Use of Force." Dr. Williams had been called to the home of a critically ill child and he tried to look in the child's throat without much success. After many trials, Dr. Williams lost his cool, became very angry, forced the child's mouth open, and saw the diphtheria-infected tonsils. He said he was so frustrated, "I could have torn the child apart with my bare hands." He had already seen two children dead in their home with diphtheria and was determined not to let it happen again. I felt the same anger, but was determined to look in the child's throat. I knew the emotion of anger was inappropriate and knew that, somehow, I needed to regain control, but the child was dying. I felt I had no choice.

With the help of the brothers, we forced the mouth open and saw the thick, green membrane blocking the child's throat. This child had diphtheria.

In a medical school lecture, one of the professors said that, in the past, diphtheria was called "the strangling angel of children" and almost all infected children died. In 1901, Emil Von Behring was presented the Nobel Prize in Medicine for developing an antitoxin for diphtheria. In 1923, an effective vaccine was developed to completely prevent the disease. With many improvements, this vaccine has been the most effective and safe preventive used in public health history. There is absolutely no reason for any child to have this horrible curse today.

This child had not been vaccinated.

The emotions of anger and disgust boiled up. How could someone allow their child to contract such a horrible condition when a preventive vaccine is readily available to everyone? The chief had told me that there are many reasons a family will take such a risk. Fear, apathy, ignorance, finances, and religious are the most common. Usually it is not a lack of knowledge but misinformation that blocks the logical and acceptable path. Even in 2015, there are families who cling to the erroneous concept that vaccines will lead to autism. These blocks to acceptable care of a child are difficult to accept. Children have a right to the best care and to avoid or ignore the best for a child is unacceptable. To me, this neglect is child abuse.

The usual course of diphtheria is coma, with death occurring within a week. Happily, this child received the diphtheria antitoxin, antibiotics, a tracheostomy, tube feedings, oxygen, and hours and hours of excellent nursing care. He survived. He spent almost a month in the hospital, with his suffering being more than any child should ever have to endure. I was worried that this child's heart may have been damaged by the diphtheria bacteria, but I never had the opportunity for follow up.

As a young physician, I felt anger and disgust toward this family and had to find a way to control these emotions. I knew that learning this control was necessary to be an effective physician. Religious beliefs are private and deeply felt, so I struggled to meet this challenge. It was critical to convince this family to get all their children vaccinated. In a quiet, soft but firm voice, just like the grandfather had used earlier, I presented the case for good medical care of their children and asked the grandfather to pray and to ask for guidance. He needed to seriously consider having all their children vaccinated immediately. The grandfather shook my hand and, after a long pause, he looked me in the eye with a steady stare and thanked me for the care of his child. Quietly, he said they would consider the advice. I felt I may not have won the war but maybe the battle.

In a large city, the children's emergency room is usually filled with families who have no regular physician and use the ER as their doctor. Frequently, they wait until the problem reaches a crisis before they go to the ER. They don't seem to mind that the building is old and been there for many years. Exam rooms are usually too small, and often crowded as entire families come together. Every room is always full of anxiety and fear.

Often, the first task is to try and relieve that anxiety. Having no idea what the weather is like outside because I had not even peeked out for the past twenty-four hours, frequently every conversation starts with "What's the weather like?" Then we go directly to the problem. With the next case, all preliminary chit-chat was unnecessary. A teen-age boy was sitting on his mother's lap and sobbing. A quick glance revealed the both sides of his face were swollen just below his ears. It was obvious this was mumps. It brought back memories of my own case of mumps when I was seven years old. My mother had given me a lemon to suck and it produced exquisite pain. This was my mother's diagnostic test for mumps. I remembered that my mumps lasted for three weeks and was a miserable experience.

The child said, "My balls hurt, so don't touch them." A complication of mumps is called orchitis, an infection and swelling of the testicles.

His mother said, "I think the mumps has gone down on him."

She was correct. His "balls" were swollen as big as golf balls and were very tender.

The mumps virus that infected his parotid glands had invaded his testicles. I told them that mumps is rarely fatal but, sadly, nothing could be done except to recommend bed rest and dreaded ice packs for his testicles. I explained to them that the child might become sterile. His testicles would heal but might shrink to the size of a pinto bean. The child apparently escaped other serious complications such as meningitis, encephalitis, and deafness.

Although mumps was first described by Hippocrates in the fifth century, it was not until 1934 that the mumps virus was discovered. Epidemics of mumps were very common among armies, and were the most common cause of deafness and meningitis during the First World War. The first mumps vaccine was developed in 1948 but had very little long-term effectiveness. It was improved and finally licensed in 1967. In 1974, it was combined with the measles and rubella vaccine and called MMR, with an effectiveness of about 90 percent with one dose and 95 percent with two. Prior to the vaccine, there were hundreds of thousands of cases every year. It was the most common cause of childhood deafness.

In the next exam room, there was a tall, thin woman holding her infant close to her breast. She was distraught, tears streaming down her pale face. She had just delivered this baby at home and the midwife told her to bring it to the emergency room immediately. Obviously, this infant was seriously damaged. The mother said the pregnancy was uncomplicated except for a rash she had when she was two months pregnant. Her other two children were sick at the same time, with German measles.

German measles is better known as rubella, or three-day measles. That is the *R* in the MMR vaccine. A mild disease in children, it is deadly to the unborn fetus when exposed in the first three months of pregnancy. At least 90 percent will develop congenital rubella. We did not know what caused this until the late 1940s, when an Australian ophthalmologist, Dr. McAlister Gregg, discovered that congenital cataracts, heart damage, brain damage, and other defects were caused by the rubella virus invading the fetus during the first trimester of pregnancy.

This little newborn suffered all of the congenital rubella complications. He emitted a high-pitched wailing cry. The examination showed he was frail, thin, and under grown. His eyes were cloudy and opacified. He was blind. A loud blowing murmur indicated the heart was damaged. I suspected deafness and seizures would develop in the near future.

Now comes the hardest part of the ER visit, as I must explain to the very upset mother that her infant is so severely damaged that there is no treatment. There is nothing that can be done. I told her that her baby would never recover and explained that his condition was caused by the German measles virus. The infant cannot be admitted to the hospital because it is still contagious and a danger to other infants and, especially, any pregnant nurses on the ward.

Sadly, the mother left with an appointment for the cardiac clinic and a heavy heart. She slowly walked away with the tiny infant wrapped in a blue blanket and clutched tightly to her breast.

CHAPTER THREE

Contagious Diseases
Pertussis, Measles

If you ever had whooping cough (pertussis), you know how miserable it can be. This disease has been preventable since 1948, but it still continues to be a problem. So many parents have neglected to immunize their children and many adults have lost their immunity. Adults with mild cases often give it to small, unvaccinated babies and children. That can be a serious problem.

A six-year-old boy named Roger was admitted to my ward with a deep hacking cough. He was in respiratory distress, and every time he tried to talk, he started coughing and could hardly get his breath. The chief of Pediatrics came into my ward with a group of medical students. As he discussed pertussis, he blew cigarette smoke into the child's face, which set off a violent spasm of coughing. The child's face became red, his eyes bulged, and out of his nose came thick, green mucus. With his inspiration, there was a loud whoop.

When he recovered, the chief said, "That, gentlemen, is a perfect demonstration of whooping cough."

It's hard to remember that smoking was so invasive in those days that no one even faulted the professor for his demonstration. (I did!) Smoking was an acceptable habit and was pervasive everywhere. I remember presenting a paper at a conference and it was hard to see my slides because of the thick cigarette smoke in the auditorium. We have known it was dangerous to our health for many years, but it has taken a long time for many people to break the addiction. I suppose the cigarette induced "whoop" was worth it and those students never forgot that sound.

Whooping cough has been described for many years. The first description was in 1578 AD. About 100 years later, the Latin word for intensive cough, *pertussis*, was introduced. The search for a prevention went on for years, with the first vaccine introduced in 1948.

Pertussis can be extremely dangerous, especially in babies and small children. There can be secondary pneumonia and, occasionally, convulsions and death. Sadly, when unvaccinated adults are infected, it is mild and rarely recognized. That is how many babies are infected.

The paradox in vaccination is that the more effective the vaccines and the gradual reduction of incidence of the disease, the more lax we become. Parents slowly lose their fear of a disease, leading to a serious number of children who are unvaccinated and susceptible. We must keep in mind that there are always individuals among society who cannot be vaccinated and who are in serious danger if they contract a disease. Individuals with cancer and the elderly and infants are especially at risk.

It is, therefore, urgent to keep the percentage of vaccinated individuals at a high level, providing what is called herd immunity. If we were able to do this, all the diseases described in this chapter would disappear from this world. It happened to smallpox and can happen to other contagious diseases.

Another preventable contagious disease is measles; the proper name is rubeola. My parents called it the "red measles." My memory of measles is still vivid because it was so miserable. My fever was high and my mother put me in a bathtub with ice water to bring it down and prevent fever seizures. The rash started in my hair and swept over my body. My father told me it would keep going down and out my toes. The red, watery eyes were the worst part of the disease. They kept my room dark because the light hurt my eyes. I coughed constantly and each cough hurt my chest. A nurse from the health department came and put a sign on our door that read "QUARANTINE – MEA-

A Child is Waiting

SLES: Do not leave or enter." I missed fifteen days of school and then my kid brother came down with measles and I missed another fifteen days.

All of this flooded my consciousness as I went into the next exam room. This little kid's eyes were bloodshot and watering. The red rash covered his head and face. The cough sounded like it came from deep in his chest. He was one miserable kid.

I looked in his mouth and saw the characteristic Koplik spots on the mucosa. These spots are like small grains of white sand surrounded by a red ring. They were first described by Dr. Henry Koplik, a New York pediatrician, and are diagnostic of measles. When I examined him, I heard mucus in his lungs and feared he was coming down with one of the dangerous complications, pneumonia. This is one of the causes of death in measles. I was also worried about encephalitis because his mother said he had been "out of his head." I remembered a lecture in medical school where the professor described a very serious complication called subsclerosing panencephalitis, a terrible sounding word meaning brain infection. The measles virus can invade any organ or area of the body and can cause appendicitis, hepatitis, and even gangrene of a foot or leg. It's rare, but it can happen.

In the past, epidemics of measles filled emergency rooms all over the country with thousands of cases. These epidemics occurred about every two to three years. In 1954, there were over 400 deaths from measles complications. When the measles vaccine was finally safe and released, these numbers dropped precipitously. Unfortunately, there is no treatment for measles. I learned that it is much better to prevent a disease than search for a treatment. Now, all we have to do is convince everyone to take advantage of these wonderful vaccines.

Perhaps it would help us understand the importance of vaccines if we reviewed history. The terrorist attack in September 2001 on the World Trade Center re-ignited the discussion of biological warfare and bioterrorism. Smallpox has been identified as a possible agent of terror.

This horrible disease was a major factor in the world for hundreds of years. We know it was present about 10,000 years ago, and Egyptian mummies show signs of the scarring. A major outbreak occurred in China in 1122 BC. In 108 AD, a smallpox epidemic, called the Antonine Plague, devastated the Roman Empire, killing almost seven million people. Actually, this was the beginning of the fall of the Roman Empire. The conquistadors introduced smallpox into the populations of the Incas and the Aztecs, devastating those cultures. It's hard to believe that the commander of the British forces suggested using smallpox against the Indians during the French–Indian war in 1754. In the 18th century, about 400,000 people died yearly from smallpox in Europe. Finally, in 1890, a Russian botanist named Dmitri Ivanovsky discovered a sub-microscopic particle that he named a *virus*, which is Latin for *toxin*. This discovery opened the door for research into discovering the cause of smallpox.

Many treatments were tried to halt the epidemics. They were all unsuccessful. Even Dr. Sydenham's prescription of "12 small bottles of beer every 24 hours" did not help. Finally, the use of variolation was tried. This consisted of injecting actual smallpox pus under the skin, and it did give immunity to those who survived the treatment.

The true breakthrough occurred when Edward Jenner, MD, a family physician, heard a milkmaid say she would never get smallpox because she had cow pox from the udders of her cows. Dr. Jenner took some of the pus from a young milkmaid, Sarah Nelms, and inoculated an eight-year-old boy, who came down with a mild case of cowpox and developed immunity to smallpox. A new and exciting preventative treatment was born. The Latin word for cow is *vacca*, and for cow pox is *vaccinia*. Dr. Jenner named this new treatment *vaccination*.

It took a while for everyone to accept this revolutionary procedure, but finally, after a worldwide epidemic occurred in 1958 in sixty-three countries, a major attack was implemented, under the leadership of the World Health Organization, to eradicate smallpox from the world. On May 8, 1980, the WHO announced that the world was free from this scourge and recommended that the practice of vaccination against smallpox be discontinued.

Children all over the world should rejoice. This attack against children and society has been conquered.

It would be wonderful if we had a vaccine to prevent premature, immature births.

CHAPTER FOUR

Prematurity

When that life-sustaining cord between mother and baby is interrupted, the very existence of the infant is at risk. The earlier in the pregnancy this occurs, the greater the risk.

I was there when a small, two-pound babe slid quietly into the harsh environment of this world. It was very early and at significant risk. Mothers are "supposed" to carry their infant for 288 days. Many pregnant women feel it's much longer than that. She must be grateful it's a relatively short time, because elephants carry their young for 640 days. Of course, a lucky house cat only carries her babes for sixty days, a kangaroo for forty days, and an opossum for twelve days.

For many reasons, frequently unknown, labor starts early and the infant comes before it is mature. If this happens before the infant has enough maturity to sustain itself, the risk becomes compounded. The organ systems are immature and do not function as efficiently as needed. This premature infant is now dependent upon all of those caregivers who are there to take the place of the mother's sustenance and to take the place of the immature organs.

I looked down at the tiny, premature infant that had just been delivered. It weighed two pounds, or 908 grams. The average infant weighs about seven pounds, or 3178 grams, at birth. In the past, physicians were taught that any infant weighing less than 1500 grams (about three pounds) would not survive and, if it did, it would be severely brain damaged or mentally retarded. We were told that an infant that small and that premature would not be "worth saving."

A Child is Waiting

When I put my hand next to this tiny infant and watched those little fingers curl around my little finger, I was awestruck by the sense of responsibility communicated by that embrace. The world of caring for premature infants has made monumental advances in the past fifty years. As I placed the infant in an ultra-modern incubator, called an isolette, I remembered the bizarre history of the development of incubators told by one of the older pediatricians.

The first warming incubators were developed in France in the 1800s. They were patterned after chick incubators. In 1886, a physician named Budin had an exhibit in the amusement section at the World's Fair in Berlin. It was set up between the yodelers and the jugglers. He set up six metal boxes with controlled heat and moisture and he called them incubators. He put small full term infants and several premature infants on display for people to pay to see. Nurses were hired to feed and care for these infants. Large crowds paid to stare at these little babies. It was a monetary success.

For the next forty years, these "incubator sideshows" continued at fairs and expositions throughout the world. In America, the first sideshow was put on display in 1898 at the fair in Omaha, Nebraska. In the Chicago World Fair in 1933–34, they were next to Sally Rand and her dancers. In 1903, an exhibit was opened in Coney Island in the "Dreamland" section. One side of the incubator was glass and the public paid ten cents to stare at these tiny babes.

This baby sideshow remained in operation until 1941. The final display was at the New York World Fair in 1939–1940. A total of ninety-six infants were exhibited during the NY Fair, with ten dying. While some died of diarrhea and infection, a mystery surrounded the other deaths. Some physicians felt it may have been due to a lack of loving warmth; as their mothers were not with them, there was an absence of maternal–infant bonding. This chapter in the lives of premature infants was colorful and interesting, but in many ways was repulsive in the exploitation of these innocent, helpless infants.

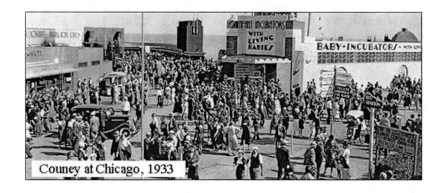

Couney at Chicago, 1933

At each World Fair and Exhibition, the incubators were improved, with constant temperature and regulated moisture, better lighting, and more glass for better visibility. Feedings and nourishment were improved. These improvements continued till the present, resulting in the modern wonderful isolettes now available in our ultra-modern Neonatal Intensive Care Units (NICU) today.

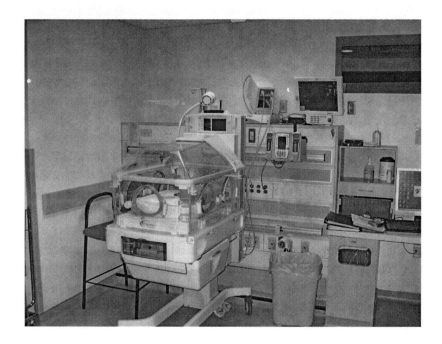

Each new invention or development slowly reduced the risk, not only for survival but for survival without damage. Respirators with pressure adapters acceptable to tiny infants, instruments built to scale, monitors to alert when an infant quit breathing, tiny needles for IV fluids, antibiotics that didn't damage the heart or kidneys, drugs to stimulate breathing and thousands of other advances aided in care.

Intensive research guided the neonatologist in deciding how much oxygen to use, how much moisture was just right, which drug did not damage, all geared toward keeping the infant alive and healthy until this little bundle of joy could handle the harsh environment beyond the womb. Some of the greatest advances have been in the development and training of physicians, nurses, respiratory therapists, and other specialized professionals who devote their lives to caring for these special infants. Learning the tricks of what works and what doesn't has been a joy to watch throughout these past twenty plus years. Many hospitals now have specialized units and a large staff of qualified and dedicated professionals whose sole job is to care for preemies, not only to see that they survive but that they survive with as minimal damage as possible. Premature infants are now transported to these NBICUs as soon as possible, often by specially equipped helicopters.

Probably the highest priority is preparing the family for the transition from the totally modern, sterile premature nursery with highly trained, skilled nurses and round the clock physicians to a loving, unskilled family. When a family is well prepared, the transition can usually result in a growing healthy infant.

The incidence of the onset of premature labor resulting in premature births has significantly increased in the past twenty years. Although the actual reasons this has happened are unknown, we know that teen pregnancy, risky lifestyles, smoking, lack of prenatal care, and poor maternal nutrition are major contributors to the problem. These attacks on the unborn infant are all preventable and treatable problems.

About four million births occur in the United States every year. Close to 15 percent (500,000) of these are premature births, defined as less than thirty-seven weeks gestation. Of these, about 5 percent (25,000) are less than two pounds, and at least 75 percent of these will survive. The daily costs in our NBICU nurseries can be rounded off at $3500 per day, often reaching one million dollars. In the last twenty years, an infant born thirteen weeks early, with a weight of two pounds and receiving special premature care has a 90 percent chance of survival.

We must also consider that, in spite of this fantastic record of survival, the incidence of significant handicapping conditions has not gone down. To date, we have not reduced the overall incidence of learning disorders, hearing and sight disorders, cerebral palsy, and a number of other disabilities. We are doing a much better job in saving infants with fewer disabilities, but there are still many factors beyond our control. The cost of managing the medical, educational, and social problems after discharge can be financially and emotionally overwhelming.

It doesn't take a genius to see that the answer to this financially overwhelming challenge to society is to reduce the number of premature births. We must reduce the onset of early labor. By seeing to it that every pregnant woman receives pre-natal care, we know we can reduce the incidence of premature births. This would be a major step in keeping these precious infants in the mother's womb until maturity. Not taking this step represents a gross failure of the political, medical, and social elements in our society. We must exert the same effort that went into the amazing improvements seen in our NBICU units.

As I looked down at that tiny bundle, I was proud to accept the responsibility of the care, attention, treatment, and love needed to see him through. The parents were constantly there to touch and hold their new son. I knew all those statistics, numbers, and predictions outlined above, but we must honor our commitment to help all children reach their highest potential. It will take a vast number of adults to accept the responsibility and see this infant to maturity and to adulthood.

CHAPTER FIVE

Newborn Screening

Every person with a new baby knows about the newborn screening heel stick done at birth. Many call it the PKU test because that is the condition (phenylketonuria) it was first used to detect, but it is now much more comprehensive than finding one single condition. This simple test can detect many problems that can attack the infant resulting in serious damage and even death. It now even includes a screening hearing test.

The dedication and commitment of a Norwegian mother, a Norwegian physician, an American microbiologist and his niece, a British mother, and a German doctor gave birth to this brain-saving procedure.

In Norway, in 1934, a mother asked a friend, Dr. Asbjorn Folling, for help. This mother told Dr. Folling that her sons, Liv, age seven years, and Dag, age four years, were retarded and their "musty" odor bothered her husband's asthma.

An inquisitive doctor, Dr. Folling started looking for the cause of the musky odor. He became excited when he found the odor was caused by a ketone called phenyl pyruvic acid in excessive amounts in the children's urine. He knew an excessive amount in the blood would damage the child's brain. Dr. Folling found several other cases and reported that it was most likely an inherited error of metabolism. He named the condition imbecillitas phenylpyruvica. He suggested a special diet of phenylalanine-free milk and food. At that time, there was none available.

In PKU, the baby inherits the gene that blocks the enzyme that is necessary to metabolize the amino acid phenylalanine to tyrosine. All milk, including breast milk, contains a significant amount of the amino acid. With the ingestion of milk, the phenylalanine builds up in the brain, causing significant damage.

In 1953, a British mother refused to accept the fact that there was no phenylalanine-free milk available for her new PKU baby. She was persistent with her doctor and, finally, Dr. Horst Bickel, a visiting German physician, took up the challenge and developed the first treatment for PKU with a phenylalanine-free special milk formula. This milk finally became commercially available in 1963.

Hopefully, parents will be told that the PKU test on their new baby is normal. If the baby has PKU that is not detected at birth and the baby starts to drink milk, disaster results.

This was the case of a family sent to me in 1966 by a family physician practicing alone in the mountains of Kentucky. This family had two retarded children and a new baby delivered at home by a midwife. The baby was six weeks old and the physician thought he was "slow." He asked me to see if I could prevent him from being retarded like his brothers. This was a tall order. The mother said, "My other two are retarded and I was hopin' you could keep this one from being the same."

When I examined the baby, he was, indeed, developmentally behind. He had poor head control, could not follow sharply with his eyes, and was extremely floppy. The laboratory studies confirmed that he had PKU (phenylketonuria). The newborn screening had not been done when he was born. The mother told me her other boys smelled "musty."

When I explained the child's problem and the treatment to the Kentucky family, they were skeptical. "But breast milk is good for you. Every baby needs milk." It was difficult, but I finally convinced them to try this new phenylalanine-free formula for several months. When they returned for a follow-up appointment, the baby was like a new child. He was smiling, cooing, attentive, and developmentally on target. Luckily, we had diagnosed the problem early enough, the new formula was available, and the family had enough trust to try it. It was too late to help her other children. This treatment is not a cure, but a method to by-pass the defect.

Genetic disease does not mean there is no treatment!

Twenty years ago, a couple in Canada were excitedly awaiting the discharge of their new baby. Their other three healthy children were at home awaiting their new brother. These parents were old hands at this. A young student nurse came into their room to review the discharge instructions. As she leafed through the chart she said, "Oh, he hasn't had his newborn screening Guthrie test. It's no big deal. I'll just stick his heel and get it done." These parents didn't know what a Guthrie test was, but a little heel stick wouldn't hurt.

Ten days later, they received a call from their doctor's receptionist. "Please bring your baby in. We want to redo the Guthrie test."

Ten days later, there was another call from the receptionist. "I'm sorry to bother you, but will you please bring your baby to the office. We want to repeat the Guthrie test again."

Ten days later, one more call from the receptionist. "You have an appointment tomorrow at 10:00 a.m. in the hospital PKU clinic. Please be on time."

PANIC!

"What is this Guthrie test? What is PKU? Why should we go? Is it serious?" They got out the encyclopedia and their lives changed forever. The book said, "Profound irreversible brain damage and mental retardation."

After a frantic phone call to the PKU clinic, the doctor gave them gentle reassurance and promised to answer all their questions at their clinic appointment, and they finally calmed down. They attended the clinic and were told their son had phenylketonuria. He was started on treatment and this young man is now a successful university student.

Luckily for thousands of infants, that's not the end of this story. This couple went on to become vigorous active advocates for neonatal screening. Their Canadian province went from newborn screening for three conditions in 2001 to screening for fifty-two conditions in 2006. This is a major accomplishment and an example of successful advocacy. This "PKU Dad" is now the volunteer treasurer for the Canadian Organization for Rare Disorders and is active in other groups.

This couple saw the problem and was willing to become part of the solution. They recognized that they had a responsibility not only to their own son but also to children all over the world. Sometimes the challenge of a life-changing event or even a disaster can result in incredible accomplishments. These accomplishments can have a significant role in improving the lives of children. Sometimes it can be a direct effect, but often it is an indirect effect.

This indirect effect occurred in the life of the author Pearl Buck. In 1920, her daughter, Carol, was born with PKU, although the condition was unknown at the time. Since the diagnosis was not known and there was no treatment, she became hopelessly retarded. As was the custom at the time, Buck was told to place her daughter in an asylum and to "forget her." To earn money to pay for this commitment, Pearl Buck wrote a book titled *The Good Earth*, and then many other successful books. She won the Pulitzer award in 1932 and the Nobel Prize for Literature in 1938. After thirty years, she finally absolved her guilt, accepted her grief, and forgave her denial. She then wrote a moving book titled *The Child Who Never Grew*. In this book, she painfully describes her desperate journey searching for answers she so urgently desired. She wrote:

> Parents may find comfort, I say, in knowing that their children are not useless, but their lives, limited as they are, are of great potential value to the human race. We learn as much from sorrow as from joy, as much from illness as from health, from handicap as from advantage- and indeed perhaps more.

Her child's unfortunate condition had provided the stimulus for Pearl Buck to utilize her God-given talent to enrich the world with her writing.

PKU is rare and many physicians will never see a case, but this genetic condition opened the door to a new and exciting procedure that has changed the lives of millions of children all over the world. It is called *newborn screening*.

To treat infants and prevent the brain damage that PKU causes, it is necessary to find it at birth or shortly afterward, and take the phenylalanine out of the diet. This led to the need for mass screening of all infants at birth. In 1957, we gave mothers a piece of filter paper to place in the infants diaper to catch the infant's urine. This was called the wet diaper test. We asked them to mail it back to us so we could analyze it for PKU. Of those sent back, many contained much more than urine and the post office complained about the smell. Many families never sent it back. This method was a complete failure.

Robert Guthrie was a microbiologist and the father of a non-PKU retarded son. His niece, Margaret Doll, was born in 1958 with PKU and became severely retarded. Her PKU was diagnosed at seventeen months of age, too late for effective treatment. One year later, Dr. Guthrie developed a simple blood test to detect PKU. This test did not need a large amount of blood. It could be done on a few drops on a piece of filter paper from a simple heel stick, as soon as the baby started drinking milk.

The simplicity of the test and the infinitesimal small cost made mass newborn screening possible. In 1963, Massachusetts became the first state to mandate, by law, that every baby have the Guthrie test for PKU. By 1970, forty-three states had enacted similar legislation, and now all states have such laws. Although not perfect, the Guthrie test serves as methodology for finding conditions at birth or shortly thereafter. Dr. Guthrie went on to refine the methodology to include a series of over thirty additional conditions, utilizing the same dried blood spots collected at birth. With the development of tandem mass spectrometry, abnormal disease components can now be detected in this simple heel stick for more than fifty disorders, and new ones are being added continually.

By discovering a condition early, it is possible for intervention and treatment to begin for many conditions, before the infant becomes affected and irreversibly damaged. Newborn screening has become more comprehensive and more successful. Since the 1970s, all states conduct newborn screening. There is, however, a wide discrepancy in the number of conditions that each state includes in the screen. In October 2005, Pennsylvania was screening for twenty-nine disorders and Texas was screening for eight. In 2006, Texas was screening for twenty-four, and many states are screening for more and more each year as knowledge, screening technologies, treatment options, and funds become available.

A worried mother brought her four-month-old son for an evaluation over the objections of the grandmother. The grandmother said, "There is nothing wrong with this baby. He is an exceptionally good baby. He's very quiet and almost never cries."

I agreed with the mother that this didn't sound right for a four-month-old. On examination, the infant was small, undergrown, developmentally delayed, and extremely floppy. A large tongue seemed to fill his mouth, the soft spot on his head was too big, and there was a protrusion through an opening in his belly button called an umbilical hernia. He was behind on all elements of the Denver Developmental Screening Test. These findings are diagnostic and often seen in a baby with congenital hypothyroidism. The laboratory tests confirmed that this was the diagnosis.

Congenital hypothyroidism, also known as cretinism, was not part of the Texas newborn screening until 1980. When the screening was started, it was found that the incidence of this disease is about 1:2500 births, and about 125 to 150 babies are found each year in Texas with a hypothyroid condition. Similar statistics have been found in other states. If this disease is treated in infants earlier than three months of age, there is a good chance the baby will develop normal intelligence, but by four months of age, he may develop a low intelligence level.

Newborn screening has become more comprehensive and more successful, making early detection and treatment a standard for every newborn. Of course, there are those who object to the extensive screening. These objections are usually based on the fear that develops when a test exposes the *risk* that a condition might develop in the future. In addition, there is always the potential for a "false positive," resulting in unnecessary worry and stress. For some conditions, there is no treatment or method of prevention. If this exists, some parents do not want to know if a condition "might" develop. All these objections are immediately rendered unacceptable when a baby is found to have a defect that is treatable, thus preventing a life-long, damaging condition.

As these tests continue to be perfected, new treatments are being discovered and preventative methods are constantly being developed. Newborn screening is a vital and critical part of the evaluation of every newborn. The Norwegian mother and doctor, the British mother and German doctor, and the American microbiologist inspired by his niece were able, by their efforts, to change the lives of millions of infants throughout the world. These individuals were willing to see the problem and use their talents to search for and find solutions. They made it possible for potentially debilitating or even life-threatening conditions to be found and treated.

●

CHAPTER SIX

Chromosomes
Down Syndrome

When I hold a new infant in the palm of my hand, I feel the potential in this new life. The sound of the first breath or the music of the first cry is like a symphony and signals an announcement that "I am here." Each newborn infant is covered with thick, slimy, offensive white mucus called vernix. When it's scrubbed off, it leaves the skin with a bright red, a warm glow that signals the potential of this new bundle of joy.

Every infant is entirely unique and I am constantly thrilled at the opportunity to be a part of this much-anticipated entrance into the world. The excitement continues as we watch the progress toward becoming a distinctive personality. We will be blessed if we are there to hear those first few words, to see those first steps, to send them off to school, and, finally, to watch the merger into adolescence and adulthood.

The greatest thrill is when I visit with a set of new parents and help them get started on the great adventure of raising a child and guaranteeing that this new life achieves the highest potential possible. Constant and continuous developmental and physical evaluations are an absolute must. We must keep in mind that one month is one half of a two-month-old infant's life.

In my mind, there is no such thing as a bad baby. When an infant is evaluated on a scale such as the Denver Developmental Screening Test, each individual element of development is examined. This includes behavioral, speech and language, and gross motor and fine motor skills. If one or more of these is incongruent with the infant's age, the task is to determine why that has occurred and if it is significant. Development is a continuous process, and though each infant is different, the process is always the same. It always goes from head to toes and from heart to fingertips. For example, an infant cannot sit alone until he holds his head up. He cannot pick up an object with his fingers until he can reach with his arms.

What if something is different or varies from the normal or the usual?

The parents must be told that their newborn infant is not perfect in all aspects. I have spent many agonizing hours searching for the best way to help parents comprehend this unexpected variation, to understand the significance, and to understand why it has happened. Their expectations of a healthy, beautiful, "perfect" infant have been building for the entire pregnancy. It becomes a challenge to help them face the reality of a different end to the pregnancy journey. The goal is to convince them that this new life they have brought into the world can be a joy, a source of happiness, and a stimulating challenge, even if it is not what they expected.

Pearl Buck, the great author and winner of the Nobel Prize for Literature, said it best in her book about her daughter who was born with PKU and was severely retarded. In her book, *The Child Who Never Grew*, she wrote:

> When your child is born to you, not whole and sound as you had hoped, but warped and defective in body or mind or perhaps both, remember, this is still your child. Remember, too, that the child has the right to life, whatever that life may be, and has a right to happiness, which you must find for him. Be proud of your child, accept him as he is, and do not heed the words and stares of those who know no better.

Parents must understand that their feelings of pain, sorrow, disappointment, guilt, and depression must be put aside, as the tiny, helpless infant in their arms will require all the strength they can muster. They must understand that it will be a challenge to their marriage, a challenge to their family, but more importantly, a challenge to each of them as individuals. If they expected a peach and received an apple, they need to realize that apple pie, baked apples, and applesauce are wonderful and can be just as good as peach pie.

One of the best examples of this happening is when a baby is born with Down syndrome.

Early one morning, I went into the nursery to see a newborn infant. This little boy was the second son of a family in my practice and they were excitedly awaiting my visit. When I held him in my arms, I knew immediately he had Down syndrome. He had all of the findings and I didn't need any special studies to confirm the diagnosis. I gathered my emotional strength and went to visit the new parents.

I said, "Your baby is healthy, but there is a problem." I explained the problem as gently as possible. The silence of disbelief was overwhelming. Finally, it was broken by the tears of anguish. Their world was changed by those few simple words.

My emotions were difficult to control, but I knew that I must. I felt their pain, their suffering, and knew that, somehow, they must be lifted out of their despair. After giving a summary of the medical details, I said, "I can assure you that this baby is going to bring joy into your life, even though you cannot see it now through your tears. He is your son and will need your love, your acceptance, and your support. Many people will be there with you, to give you guidance, hope, and encouragement at every step of the way. There will be people who stare and still use the term 'Mongoloid' but you must ignore them."

This distasteful name started when the characteristics were first described in 1866 by Dr. John Langdon Down. Dr. Down published a paper in England, where he described a set of retarded children who were in a mental asylum near London, where he was the superintendent. The paper was titled "Observations on an Ethnic Classification of Idiots." The paper described children that had features that resembled the Mongoloid race and were retarded. Dr. Down called them Mongoloids because he assumed that the darker the skin, the more feebleminded a person, so he based his classification of retardation on racial and ethnic characteristics.

It's hard to believe that it took 100 years for this greatly mistaken assumption to be openly challenged. In the early 1960s, the Asiatic Genetic Researchers challenged this idea and the term Mongolian Idiots was dropped and changed to Down syndrome.

The mother fearfully asked, "How did this happen? Was it something I did or something I didn't do?"

I explained to the parents that, in 1959, the cause of Down syndrome was found to be an abnormality with the chromosomes. In the human body, each cell contains twenty-three pairs of chromosomes, for a total of forty-six. Twenty-two of these pairs, called autosomes, are virtually alike.

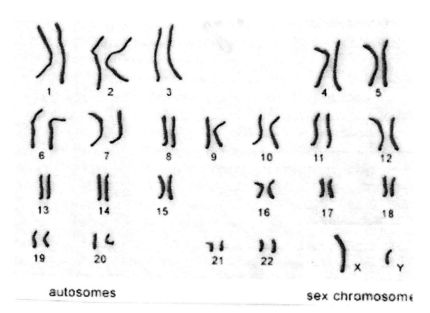

The 23rd pair is called the sex chromosome and determines the baby's sex. Females have a pair of X chromosomes and males have one X and one Y. Every living plant and animal has a set of chromosomes in each cell that determine who or what they will be. A fruit fly has only eight pairs, a house cat has thirty-eight, a guinea pig has sixty-four; all compared to the human, who has forty-six. There are thousands of genes on each chromosome. In the case of Down syndrome, when the cells are formed, the 21st chromosome contains three instead of a pair. This abnormality is then repeated in every cell in the body. This extra set of genes results in all of the symptoms and signs we see in this developmental problem. The condition is properly called trisomy 21.

One of our first goals is to counter the guilt and blame that will interfere with parents accepting reality. Inevitably, parents will ask the same questions. "What did I do to cause this?" "Should I have taken more vitamins?" "I told my wife she should exercise more." "Maybe it is due to my drinking." "Did the marijuana I smoked in college cause this to happen?"

They always seem to blame themselves. I explain that it was not their fault and that it was nothing they did or didn't do. We do not know why this happens. It is a chance occurrence.

There is no place for guilt or blame. Those feelings are serious impediments to clear and productive action. Hopefully, the parents can understand how this unfortunate condition developed and, therefore, eliminate the guilt and the blame. They must concentrate on the present and on what they can do.

Another difficult emotion frequently expressed is denial. Sometimes this is hard to confront and acceptance of the truth depends upon them working through the denial that is almost always present. "I can see his eyes are shaped differently, but my uncle has eyes just like that." "His ears are shaped like his grandmother's ears." "Those short stubby fingers are like my great aunt."

With careful and clear explanations, denial can usually be eased to the background and the parents and the extended family can finally begin to face their challenge.

Finding someone with experience working with children with various developmental problems can be helpful. Those of us who have lived through this experience, and many parents who have, can truthfully point out how wonderful, loving, and pleasant this little baby can be. He will bring joy into their lives.

Sure, it will be work, it will require patience, and it will require understanding. Sometimes, it will be a battle to get the very best for him. With all of the adults in this child's life working together, this child can be brought to his greatest potential. The challenge often brings growth in all who face it.

Dr. Craig Ramey, in his book, *Right from Birth*, put it this way:

> The challenges and uncertainties of parenting won't go away, but the rewards can be greater the more you appreciate the amazing accomplishments of your baby's total development, the more you understand the lasting importance of the love and support you provide, and the more you delight in your child's uniqueness, right from birth.

I remember one infant with Down syndrome who was completely accepted by his parents. They fought continually to see that his rights were assured, and he is now is a senior in high school, where he is accepted and loved by all of his classmates.

Another of my children was a delightful child with Down syndrome who also became a joy to her family. One day, when she had become a young woman, she came up to me in a local store. I had been her pediatrician throughout most of her life and we were good friends. She was excited to see me and gave me a big hug.

She excitedly said, "Dr. James, I have a job." I was proud of her and told her so.

She proudly said, "And I have benefits!"

Her mother told me she had worked for Prudential Insurance Company for two years and never missed a day of work. She was a loyal, dedicated employee. This family had convinced this young lady she could do anything she set her heart to accomplish. She had lived up to her potential, even though it was limited. I was honored to have been a part of this family. I was honored to be her friend. This represents the best of parenting.

Recently, I was in a class learning how to set up a blog. One of the students was a teen-aged boy with Down syndrome.

It was a joy to watch him learn to set up his personal blog and write the first paragraph of his planned weekly blog.

My philosophy has always been that if we can help children with limitations live up to 80 percent of their abilities, they will equal or surpass those without limitations who only live up to 10 percent of theirs.

Whenever a child develops a serious problem, immediately everyone begins a search for the cause and the cure. If someone has the knowledge of the cause, is willing to spend the time helping the parents comprehend what has happened, and the parents are willing to listen, the results can be rewarding for all concerned.

What if the cause is not known? What happens then? If the cause is not known, there is usually no cure and, frequently, there may be only minimal treatment. I have watched this in many families and it is like a steamroller. Blame, guilt, anger, denial, and depression intrude into their lives. These and many other emotions become so important that, often, the child and his condition are completely forgotten and ignored.

The trisomy of Chromosome 21 occurs about 1:700 pregnancies and is the most common chromosomal defect. Other trisomies are trisomy 18 (Edward syndrome) and trisomy 13 (Patau syndrome). These defects are associated with multiple congenital malformations and are usually not compatible with life beyond the first few months. Other trisomies usually result in the fetus being aborted (miscarried) in the first month or so in pregnancy.

Our society is so tuned to quick fixes for our problems that it is hard to accept the concept that there may be no "fix." So often we go to our physician "for a shot" for whatever "ails us." Those days when we sat by the bedside and held the hand of a child with polio, cystic fibrosis, or diphtheria, knowing there was nothing that could be done, are so easily forgotten. That there is "nothing we can do to cure your child" is not an acceptable answer, even if it's the truth. Perhaps the best solution to the frustration that parents and professionals frequently feel is to recognize and face the problem as soon as possible, to apply the answers we know to be correct, avoiding pure conjecture, to search for new solutions, and to find the power and energy necessary to never stop.

Every infant should expect no less.

CHAPTER SEVEN

Genes

Fragile X, Angelman Syndrome, Prader-Willi Syndrome

There has been a total explosion of information about our molecular structure. The research into our chromosomes and genes has brought a complete revision of our thinking as to how we become who we are. The Human Genome Project has identified and plotted a huge number of the genes that each of us has received from our parents, our grandparents, and ancestors. Scientists have identified thousands of genetic differences that result in attacks on the "normal" outcome of the joining of the ovum and sperm to give birth to a human being.

The most common hereditary cause of mental disability in boys is the Fragile X syndrome. It occurs in about 1:4000 males and in 1:8000 females. Males have more severe symptoms than females. These children experience a range of developmental and learning problems.

When I first saw Mike, he was in kindergarten and just could not learn. He had a short attention span, problems relating to other children, a slight stutter, significant anxiety, and he disliked being touched. His physical exam revealed a high arched palate, a high forehead, and prominent ears. His head was larger in relationship to his body. He had been diagnosed as autistic, with ADHD, MR, anxiety disorder, and several others. Multiple medications had been tried with no positive effect. The year was 1991 and the gene for Fragile X had just been identified. It was named the *Fragile X mental retardation 1 gene* (FMR1). Mike and I were lucky enough to have his karyotype run and it was positive for Fragile X.

The fragile X gene consists of a fragile mutation site on the X chromosome, causing a constriction. This constriction results in the FMR1 protein not being produced. When this protein is deficient, a number of abnormalities occur. The broad spectrum of problems is the result of a various level of this deficiency. The range is from severe mental deficiency to a state of normal cognitive ability but with behavioral problems and learning problems. Mike was a typical child with Fragile X. The mother reported he had been slow in language development early in life. His hyperactivity complicated the picture.

By making the proper diagnosis, it was now possible to plan an educational program appropriate for his level of ability, to try appropriate medications, and to recognize that this is a genetic disorder and not just a bad kid acting out.

Girls can have Fragile X syndrome, but usually are not as severely affected. This is because females have two X chromosomes, and the fragile X defect is present on only one of the X chromosomes. The second X chromosome acts as a buffer and helps reduce the symptoms. Girls who are affected usually have attentional problems, disorganized behavior, and speech problems.

Another major problem can occur when a deficient gene just doesn't function. This is often called a deletion, as if it were not even there. When a gene is absent or not functioning, disaster occurs.

Jacqueline was a beautiful baby.

She was the second child of a family whose parents were studying to become teachers. They were not prepared for the challenge that was about to turn their life upside down. The mother had been exceptionally careful during pregnancy. No smoking, no drinking, exercise, good food, plenty of rest, and everything she could think of to have a healthy pregnancy. There was no history of congenital defects in their family. As the second child of teachers, Jackie was constantly tested by her parents. At six months of age, her mother was taking a class in child development and she felt Jackie was not developing as she should. In spite of reassurances from everyone, the mom enrolled her in an early infant development program. She needed to find out why this beautiful little girl was not doing well. It is always imperative to find out the why and what before jumping into a treatment program that could even make things worse.

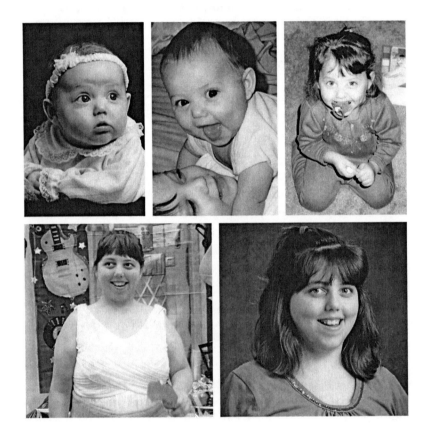

Jacqueline's chromosomes revealed a major defect on the 15th chromosome. On the 15th chromosome, there is a particular set of genes that control the function and production of a protein called ubiquitin. This protein is responsible for brain growth and function. It is called the UBE3A gene, and is located on the maternal 15th chromosome. Without the function of the gene and, therefore, the absence of this protein, parts of the brain do not develop as they should. An analysis of body cells for the chromosomes can identify this defect.

In 1964, a pediatrician named Harry Angelman lived in Warrington, England. Three children were admitted to his ward with similar characteristics. They had inappropriate smiles and laughter in addition to being significantly developmentally delayed. He did not know the cause of their problem. When he was on holiday in Verona, Italy he saw a painting titled *The Boy with a Puppet*. The laughing face of the puppet reminded him of those children. In 1965, he published a paper that he titled "The Happy Puppet Children." That name stuck and children with the same characteristics as he described were called Happy Puppet Children. Finally, in 1987, the name of the syndrome was changed to Angelman syndrome. He described a group of children who had protruding tongues, jerky movements, and curious bouts of laughter. We know now that these findings are neurogenetic, which means the genes affect the brain and nervous system. These children often have seizures, developmental delay, mental retardation, speech impairment, difficulty with coordination and balance, and behavior difficulties.

Due to the generalized nature of this syndrome, children are often misdiagnosed. The Angelman Syndrome Foundation has developed a checklist of symptoms to look for.

- In infants 0 to twenty-four months: A lack of cooing or babbling, inability to support the head, cannot pull oneself to standing, delayed motor skills
- In children older than twenty-four months: A lack of speech or a delay in speech, delayed ability to walk, unstable gait or balance issues
- Seizures often begin at between two and three years of age.
- An inappropriately happy demeanor, frequent laughing, smiling, and excitability

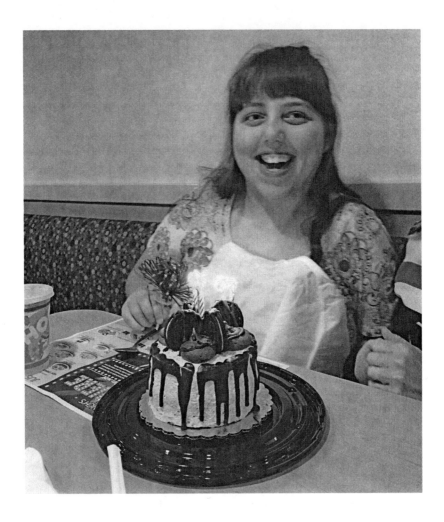

Jackie had most of these problems. Angelman syndrome is rare, occurring in about one in 15,000 births. To these worried parents, it was not rare. It presented a major challenge. To help Jackie's teachers understand the problem, Jackie's mom, a very intelligent woman, developed a PowerPoint presentation and, every year, presented it to Jackie's new teachers and to her new classmates. This helped everyone understand why Jackie acted in her own difficult way. These parents have included Jackie in as many experiences as she can tolerate. She has now passed twenty years old and is still an integral part of the family in spite of her limitations.

Another example of genes that are not functioning is the Prader-Willi syndrome. While the gene for Angelman syndrome is carried by the mother, a similar defect in the same region on chromosome 15 is carried by the father. This defect consists of non-functioning genes in the 15q11-13 area. This syndrome was first reported in 1956, with infants presenting with low muscle tone (hypotonia), poor suck, and failure to thrive. At around two years, the hypotonia improves, but the child develops insatiable appetite and soon becomes obese. Several features develop, including undescended testicles, small hands and feet, short stature, small penis, and mental retardation.

The newest research is targeted toward finding a way to turn on the non-functioning genes. If this could be done early enough in the child's development, perhaps the brain could be stimulated to develop normally. The research is not there yet, but it is exciting to consider the possibilities. With early diagnosis, tailored interventions can certainly help these children reach their maximum potential.

Whenever a child is found to be delayed in any developmental milestone, the first question to answer is whether it is a normal variation or a sign of abnormality. If there is a suspicion of abnormality, an extensive search for the cause should begin immediately. In almost every occasion, early diagnosis results in better outcome.

CHAPTER EIGHT

Congenital Defects
Spina Bifida, Hydrocephalus

The brain and spinal cord are the most sensitive and vital parts of the human body. When something goes wrong with either of these critical organs, it takes the combined knowledge of a group of therapists, the bravery of a child, and the patience and dedication of parents to find a way to manage this challenge. Spina bifida and hydrocephalus require all the effort we can expend.

The fashion show for special needs children was sponsored by the Spina Bifida Association. It was held in the auditorium at Morgan's Wonderland in San Antonio, Texas. Hundreds of chairs were filled with a large number of advocates, who were enthusiastic and dedicated to these special children. There were grandparents, aunts, uncles, and a lot of friends. High school design students from three local high schools had designed and tailored unique outfits for each special needs child. Young teen volunteers helped guide them on the stage and family members filled the auditorium at Morgan's Wonderland with cheers and applause. The special children just glowed with excitement as they modeled their new outfits. There were various disabilities among those present, including spina bifida, Down syndrome, cerebral palsy, autism, brain damage, Angelman syndrome, and others.

Patiently sitting in a chair, waiting her turn to model her new outfit, was one of the most beautiful teen-aged girls I had ever seen. Her dazzling smile was like a magnet and drew people to her. She was made up with a bit of rouge on her cheeks, a faint glow of lipstick, and perfectly arched eyebrows. Tiny gold earrings sparkled, and a ribbon in her perfectly coiffured hair completed the picture. When they called her name, she struggled with her crutches and slowly moved toward the stage on legs that had lost their purpose. Her curved spine kept her from standing upright, but she held her head high. Her lovely smile greeted the audience, who cheered and shouted in appreciation of the confidence and pride that she radiated. Her spina bifida had robbed her of her ability to walk and of a healthy body, but nothing was going to rob her of her fearless spirit.

Spina bifida is the most commonly occurring permanently disabling birth defect in the United States. It occurs in the first month of pregnancy. In the normal process of growth and development of the fetus, the spinal cord is open and gradually closes, forming a tube that is then covered by the spinal bones. If the spine fails to close, it is called spina bifida. Many of these cases are minor and do not affect the infant, but if the spinal nerves are damaged, a severe disability occurs. The results are a lack of feeling in the body from the defect down, a partial paralysis with a loss of use of the legs, and problems with bladder and bowel control. The spine may not grow normally, resulting in a curved spine called scoliosis.

The Spina Bifida Association estimates that there are over 166,000 individuals in the US with this defect. Soon after the baby is born, the child and parents must work intensely with occupational therapist and physical therapist. The earlier the therapy begins, the better the outcome. This therapy continues as the child starts to school and has the benefit of a well-trained special educational teacher and exposure to the social interaction of other children.

The exact cause of this sometimes devastating condition has not been discovered. The most important fact that all 65 million women of child bearing age in this country must learn is that the risk of spina bifida can be reduced by 70 percent by the simple task of taking 400 micrograms of folic acid every day.

Think about it! Since the cause is unknown, every woman is at risk of a spina bifida pregnancy. The defect occurs in the first month, before most women even know they are pregnant, but by taking a single dose of folic acid every day, starting before getting pregnant, that risk is significantly reduced. It is certainly worth the effort.

Another problem that can damage the central nervous system is hydrocephalus. It can occur with spina bifida, but there are many other causes that must be investigated. As a medical student at the University of North Carolina, one of my rotations was through the North Carolina State Hospital in Goldsboro, NC. It was there I saw my first baby with hydrocephalus. The word comes from the Greek *hydro*, which means water, and *cephalus*, which means head. Hydrocephalus has been called "water on the brain," although the water is actually cerebrospinal fluid.

Even though Hippocrates first described hydrocephalus many centuries ago, no successful preventive treatment has been developed. The babies in the state hospital had heads larger than basketballs. They couldn't even turn over due to the weight and size of their heads. They would kick their legs, wave their arms, and smile. As I moved from one side of the crib to the other, they would try valiantly to turn their heads, but could not. The caretakers would prop their bottles on pillows so they could nurse. I was haunted by their eyes, where the whites were prominent above the pupils. I was told this is called "sunset eyes" and is a sure sign of hydrocephalus. Some of the children became blind.

I asked the hospital staff what treatments were available. They told me the only one available at that time was to insert a needle through the brain into the cavities, called ventricles, and draw off the fluid. When that was done, the head would collapse, like letting air out of a ball. If the baby didn't die from this treatment, the fluid and pressure would just return. These fragile infants desperately needed someone to accept the challenge and develop an acceptable treatment.

Ten years later, a six-week-old infant was lying quietly on my exam table. She was smiling, cooing, and acting like any other six-week-old, but her head was noticeably larger than it should be, measuring above the 90th percentile. The bones, called skull plates, surrounding her brain were widely separated and the soft spot was bulging. She kicked her legs, moved her arms, and looked at me with clear, alert eyes, but could not lift that heavy head. The white portion of the eyes could be seen above the pupils.

The mother anxiously asked, "What's wrong with my baby? What has happened? Her head is too big."

I explained that there are cavities in the brain called ventricles where cerebrospinal fluid is constantly being produced. Under normal circumstances, these ventricles fill with the fluid, and then drain through a small canal down into the spinal space and around the spinal cord, where the fluid is absorbed into the body rather than being lost. About two cups are made each day. If that fluid is lost, the baby will soon become seriously dehydrated. As the fluid is made constantly, when that canal is blocked by a congenital defect such as spina bifida, trauma, bleeding, tumor, or infection, the pressure builds up in the ventricles and the head enlarges. In infants, the skull plates have not grown together, so the head enlarges as the skull plates separate, which prevents a rapid increase in pressure within the brain. This condition occurs in about one infant in a thousand births.

A regular X-ray does not show the ventricles, and such miraculous machines as CT scans, MRIs, or ultra-sound had not yet been invented. We had to get air into these cavities to provide a contrast before the X-ray of the skull would reveal their size. To do this required a distasteful procedure that was necessary. While someone held the baby's head upright, I anesthetized the skin, and inserted a long needle through the soft spot on the top of the head down through the brain and into the ventricle. After withdrawing some of the spinal fluid, I injected air, which produced a large bubble in the ventricle. Then, carefully holding the head upright, we shook the head to get the bubble to go to the top and hoped a seizure didn't occur. We took the child to X-ray and the picture showed enlarged ventricles, clearly outlined by the contrast between the air bubble and the brain. This was diagnostic of hydrocephalus.

In the early 1950s, an innovative and courageous neurosurgeon named Eugene Spitz developed a new procedure where a polyethylene tube was inserted into the ventricle, then threaded under the skin, and the fluid was diverted around the blocked canal and into the abdominal cavity or the heart. This relieved the pressure; the fluid was not lost. It was called a ventriculoperitoneal shunt. This procedure used a very expensive valve that was only marginally effective as a pressure regulator in an effort to keep the pressure in the brain constant.

A person does not have to be a physician, a scientist, or professional to improve the lives of children. One only has to be willing to see the problem and love children enough to accept the challenge to find the answer. The contribution of two fathers whose sons had hydrocephalus would change the lives of these unfortunate children. They saw the problem in their own sons and found a way to solve it.

John Holter was an industrial machinist. Casey, his son, was born in November 1955. Casey was born with a congenital blockage of the outflow of his spinal fluid from the brain. This blockage resulted in hydrocephalus. John was afraid of the repeated needle taps of the brain that were being used to release the pressure. The neurosurgeon inserted a tube to drain the fluid but the valve to regulate the pressure was continually becoming obstructed. Even though he knew little about medicine, Holter put his ingenuity and mechanical knowledge to work to solve the problem by designing a new one-way pressure valve to be used on his son. This new Holter valve was a significant improvement over the old one and a lifesaving breakthrough for babies with hydrocephalus. The Holter valve is still used today.

Unfortunately, Casey developed a reaction to the polyethylene tube used to drain the fluid. Again, Holter went to work and invented a new material that he named silastic. A combination of silicone and rubber, this new material did not produce a rejection reaction in the body. A tube made of silastic was used in his son. Today, it is used extensively in heart valves, breast implants, and many other medical interventions.

Another father, Roald Dahl, was a poet and author of many children's stories, including *Willy Wonka and the Chocolate Factory*, *James and the Giant Peach*, and *Matilda*. When his son Theo was four months old, his carriage was struck by a taxi, causing a bleed into his brain that resulted in a blockage and hydrocephalus. The Holter valve that was used to relieve the pressure kept getting obstructed, causing the pressure to build up in the brain, resulting in seizures. Dahl was not an engineer, but he had a powerful imagination, along with being pragmatic and resourceful. He utilized that imagination and revised the Holter valve into a new "constant pressure" valve that was almost free from obstruction. It saved his son's life.

The intense emotional involvement, the constant fear for their sons, and the courage to step out stimulated these fathers to solve the problem presented to them. Their advocacy made it possible to relieve the pressure causing hydrocephalus in millions of children. My little patient received the Spitz procedure using the silastic tube and the Dahl-adapted Holter valve. He did extremely well. Untreated, these babies will become blind, severely retarded, and gradually lose their brain tissue. The future of my patient and millions of other affected children is brighter because of the contributions of those two fathers.

Children with hydrocephalus who are diagnosed early and receive acceptable treatment can avoid many of the central nervous problems that interfere with good daily functioning.

CHAPTER NINE

Genetic Defect
Cystic Fibrosis

Every cell in the body has a set of genetic information. Included in the genes, this set of instructions tells the body how to develop, how to function, and how to make this living creature unique. These genes are responsible for making certain proteins that regulate growth and development and physical appearances like hair color, etc. All this information is stored in the genes on the chromosomes as DNA (deoxyribonucleic acid). There are variants in the DNA in all of us, because we receive DNA from each parent. We end up different from our parents, though a combination of both. If we receive the same information from both parents, that characteristic will be expressed in our body.

Occasionally, there can be a mutation or a change in a gene that can spell disaster in our lives. An example of this is seen in a condition called cystic fibrosis.

One night, an underweight, under-grown, emaciated nine-year-old child named Harlan was brought in from the surrounding Kentucky hills in critical condition. His grandmother said, "That child is going to strangle to death if you don't do something."

She fearfully told me that his forehead tasted salty when she kissed him. She knew an old adage imported to this country from northern Europe: "Woe to the child which, when kissed on the forehead, tastes salty. He is bewitched and soon must die."

Harlan had cystic fibrosis. A diagnosis can be made when there is a high salt content in sweat. It was the 1960s and the sweat test to measure salt content was the gold standard for the diagnosis. In fact, it was the only test we had available. Harlan was terminally ill. We placed him in an oxygen tent full of mist, started an IV with antibiotics, and tried to help him cough up globs of thick green mucus by clapping on his back, in an effort to stave off the death that seemed to be inevitable. All treatments were fruitless and he continued to go downhill.

As his doctor and his advocate, it was frustrating to be unable to do more to relieve his suffering. On his third night, I was sitting by his bedside doing the only thing I could do to make his life more bearable, reading him a story.

He loved the story of *James and the Giant Peach*. Harlan looked at me with sad, piercing eyes, as only a nine-year-old can, and asked, "Am I going to die?"

I was startled! How honest could I be? How honest should I be? I looked at his blue lips and gray complexion. I felt his faint, rapid pulse and looked at his blue, clubbed fingers. He was struggling to breathe.

"Yes, you are going to die, but I don't know when."

"Will it be tonight?"

"Maybe."

"I thought so. Will you hold me till it happens?"

Without hesitation, I crawled into the tent and held him close to my chest for an hour or so. He held on to me until his breathing stopped and his pounding heart raced no more. He looked so peaceful when the struggle was finally over. In spite of my tears, I realized at that moment that sometimes death can be a blessing

I am grateful to tell you, things have changed.

We have learned so much about cystic fibrosis and our treatments have significantly improved, so that the life expectancy has now improved. For a child born in 2010 with CF, the life expectancy is thirty-seven years for females, and forty years for males. In 1966, the CF Foundation started a registry, gathering data on 26,000 CF patients. In those early days, death could be blamed on malnutrition. As we learned more, we were able to improve the nutritional status of these children. We then targeted the respiratory system with intensive research and new treatments. With all of that, the lives of these children began to improve and we began to add years to their longevity.

Perhaps the greatest breakthrough came with the genetics revolution. CF is due to an autosomal recessive mutation in the genetic coding for the CF transmembrane conductance regulator protein (CFTR). This gene is located on the long arm of human chromosome 7. Both parents must carry this gene for the infant to have CF. If both parents are carriers, there is a 1 in 4 chance with every pregnancy that the offspring will have cystic fibrosis. It is the most common lethal genetic disease in the Caucasian population. It exists in Hispanics and African Americans, but is rare in the Oriental population. To date, 1864 different mutations have been described on chromosome 7. Simply speaking, there is a disruption in the normal, well-balanced flow of sodium and chloride (salt) with fluid through the cell walls of the body. The faulty expression of the CFTR gene in the airways and lungs, the intestines, pancreatic ducts, bile ducts, vas deferens, and sweat glands result in the disease manifestations. These mutations result in a thick mucus obstructing the passages in multiple organs.

The 1864 mutations could be broken down into six classes. Each class has a unique effect on the cell and the electrolyte and fluid balance. Research has now begun to target each class of mutation to find a method to reverse the mutation or at least improve it to become more functional. Some could even possibly restore function to the CFTR mutant gene. Cystic fibrosis is the first human genetic disease to benefit from the recent advances in genetic engineering. The development of three animal (pigs, mice, and ferrets) models with CFTR mutations have greatly increased the possibility of finding new and exciting treatments.

The G551D CFTR mutation is in the second class of the mutations. With significant support from the CF Foundation, clinical research was conducted by Vertex Pharmaceuticals, and a new drug named Ivacaftor was discovered to be effective in reversing the effects of this specific mutation. After several studies were performed showing positive results, this drug was FDA-approved for CF patients who had this specific mutation.

It is marketed under the name Kalydeco. This drug and several others have been designed to work at the site of the basic defect. In CF the "gates" at the cell level do not open and allow the proper movement of chloride across the cell membrane. This results in the thick mucus that blocks various organs, especially the lungs. These new drugs are designed to open those "gates."

The FDA has now approved Kalydeco for eight additional mutations of the CFTR gene. In June 2014, Vertex reported a new study in *Medscape*. In this study, Kalydeco was used in combination with an experimental drug called lumacaftor in CF patients with the F508del mutation. The results are promising and Vertex requested FDA approval for this treatment. In May 2015, the FDA advisory committee recommended approval for this new drug.

All this wonderful new progress would not be possible without the financial support of the CF Foundation AND the willingness of many CF patients and their families to volunteer and participate in the research. It takes a strong individual to be part of a trial of an unknown drug. These brave patients and their parents are to be complimented for this effort.

The median age of diagnosis for CF children is six to eight months, but this may improve with more newborn screening and more genetic testing.

Cystic Fibrosis is characterized by:

- Chronic obstruction and infection of the respiratory tract
- Pancreatic insufficiency with poor nutrition
- Elevated sweat chloride levels

The earliest clinical manifestation of pancreatic insufficiency in some patients is meconium ileus in the newborn infant. A thick, black mucoid material called meconium blocks the intestine. It frequently requires surgery for correction if it cannot be relieved with a Gastrografin enema. This obstruction can even be found before birth. About 16 to 20 percent of CF infants will have meconium ileus. It can occur in infants without CF.

Other complications include gastroesophageal reflux, which will further complicate the respiratory problems. Biliary tract disease, with blockage of the digestive enzymes from the pancreas, results in the loss of large amounts of fat in the stool, carrying with it vital nutrients. The resulting malnutrition can be extremely serious. By taking large amounts of digestive enzymes, the malnutrition can be prevented. Gall bladder abnormalities, even with gallstones, are a rare but bothersome complication. About 22 percent of CF children will suffer from rectal prolapse.

Medical management of CF has three main goals:

- Control respiratory infections and clearing the airways of the thick mucus
- Provide intensive nutritional therapy with enzyme and mineral supplements, including multivitamins. This should maintain adequate growth and nutrition. It is important to report that a research project reported at the European Cystic Fibrosis Society in 2015 revealed that infants started on a fortified breast milk formula or a high-density formula showed significantly improved nutritional status. This is a proven reason for early diagnosis.
- Manage all the complications as soon as they occur

Delayed puberty and reduced fertility are usually present. Most CF males are azoospermatic due to the lack of development of the vas deferens in the testicles. CF females are usually fertile and many successful pregnancies have been reported.

Cystic fibrosis is a serious disease and if untreated will always result in an early death. Children with CF have benefited from the intensive research that has been carried out all over the world. The new field of genetic therapy has demonstrated the exciting future, not only in CF but in the possibilities that exist for other diseases.

This brings up a serious but necessary dilemma. Is it ethical for us to manipulate these building blocks of our actual humanity? If we can manipulate genes—change them, delete them, substitute other genes in their place, turn them on or turn them off—do we have a right to do this, or should we? Perhaps we should ask the cystic fibrosis patients for their opinion.

The miraculous development of these new drugs has created an ethical and financial dilemma. The cost of development for pharmaceutical companies is extremely high. This causes the drugs to be extremely expensive and beyond the financial resources of many families. Insurance companies and government medical programs are faced with this unexpected cost. Yet, the drugs are critical for many CF patients. We must find an answer to this grave equation. As new and wonderful drugs are developed for many other conditions, this same problem is going to exist. Perhaps it is time for all concerned to begin a dialogue to find an acceptable solution. I recommend that all parents begin this dialogue with their insurance company and with their elected government representatives as soon as possible.

CHAPTER TEN

Prenatal Attacks
AIDs, CMV, Rh Factor

The protection the unborn child receives while in the womb can be broken down if the mother is attacked by infections, by drugs, or, actually, by anything that affects the mother. This may be through the blood stream across the placenta to the infant, in the amniotic fluid surrounding the baby, via direct infection during the birth process, or even through the breast milk. Often the results of these attacks can have devastating consequences.

Molly came to see me two weeks before her due date. She was extremely upset, agitated, and depressed. Through her sobs, she told me she was HIV positive and she was eight months pregnant. Her distress was for her unborn baby. She told me her ELISA test and her western blot assay were both positive. "What does this mean?" she sobbed.

Gently, I explained that the human immunodeficiency virus (HIV) could have entered her body through unprotected sex with an infected person, through sharing needles or other drug paraphernalia, or through an infected blood transfusion. All blood is tested for HIV in the United States, and she had not been transfused. Since the HIV virus cannot live outside the body, it cannot be spread by kissing or drinking after an infected person, or from contact with saliva, sweat, tears, urine, feces, or insect bites. It is spread in vaginal fluid, semen, blood, or in breast milk. It can affect the baby in the birth process or it can infect the baby after birth through breast milk.

A Child is Waiting

Once in the body, the HIV virus attacks and destroys the white blood cells known as CD4+. These cells are part of the body's immune system that fights off infection and disease. When the immune system is destroyed or even weakened, it allows certain illnesses, such as specific types of pneumonia and cancer, to attack the body. When this happens, it is called Acquired Immune Deficiency Syndrome (AIDS).

I explained to Molly that we can usually prevent the baby from contracting the virus by treating the mother with medication before delivery and the baby after birth. I cautioned her that she must not breastfeed her baby. At that time, the current treatment drug was ZDV. It was very expensive, so I gave her the name of a local AIDS clinic where she could be treated for free. We called, made an appointment, and sent her to the clinic. If I had known what was going to happen, I would have driven her there myself.

She disappeared, and the next time I saw her was five months later. She appeared in my office with the sickest little four-month-old infant I had ever seen. The pressure of testing positive for HIV had been too much for her and she had relapsed into her previous drug addicted state. The drugs robbed her of the ability to make good decisions for herself and, more importantly, for her baby. She had not gone to the clinic and had not been treated. She delivered an HIV positive infant.

Now, at four months of age, the infant was developing AIDS. I called an AIDS clinic and had my nurse personally take her and the baby to the clinic. This beautiful, innocent little child may not live with the triple burden of AIDS, poverty, and a parent who is addicted, infected, and dying.

AIDS is truly a worldwide pandemic. It is one of the most difficult medical challenges facing society today. Since the HIV virus first made a known appearance in our society, it has become the leading cause of death worldwide. The first known cases were reported in 1970, but by 1980, it was present on five continents. In 1981, the CDC reported on the first cases of Kaposi sarcoma (KS) and Pneumocystis carini (PC) caused by the HIV virus. In July 1982, there were only 452 cases reported in the US, but by1984, there were 7,699 cases and 3665 deaths. In 2005, there were 3.1 million known worldwide deaths from AIDS. Over half a million were children. In 2005, we knew of over 700,000 new cases in children under fifteen years of age. Due to under-reporting, there are probably many more than that. Most of these children became infected during childbirth or from breastfeeding. Up to 60 percent of infants who become infected from their mothers die before two years of age. The number of children orphaned from parental AIDS is staggering.

Molly and her baby are lucky because they live in one of the First World countries where new treatment is becoming available on a regular basis. Funding, trained professionals, and resources are available for her and her baby. With all these resources, they might live. In many other places in the world, the countries are the "have-nots" and there are minimal resources available.

There has been a major effort by many countries throughout the world to combat this menace to mankind. In the US government, a number of federal agencies are participating in the fight, including the Department of State, Department of Health and Human Services, the CDC, the FDA, the HRSA Global HIV/AIDS program, NIH, and many others. In addition, there are many private organizations in the US that have dedicated millions in resources in this critical fight. The most prominent ones include the Global Fund to Fight Aids, The International Aids Society, the Kaiser Family foundation, UNAIDS, and WHO. New drugs are constantly being developed and a vaccine seems to be almost certain in the near future.

In spite of all this effort, the epidemic continues, although the pace has slowed. Once infected, the semen, vaginal fluid, and blood are always infectious, even with treatment. These are frightening conditions for the continuation of a worldwide epidemic. The unchecked spread of the disease from those first few reported cases in 1972 to the epidemic we see today is a dramatic warning to the entire world. It is clear that, with education, prevention, and treatment, this plague on mankind can be checked. Our citizens must recognize that a devastating epidemic in a faraway place in the world will, sooner or later, affect them. They must accept the responsibility of helping their fellow human beings. It has happened in the past with other diseases and challenges and, maybe, just maybe, this challenge of HIV/AIDS will be conquered. It will take the acceptance that our society has a responsibility toward those who are suffering throughout the world.

There are other infections that can affect the unborn infant. One of the most common is the cytomegalovirus (CMV).

There is a sign in the lobby of Texas Children's Hospital in Houston that reads, "The most common virus that people never heard of. In Texas, a newborn baby dies from CMV infection every nine days. In Texas, a newborn baby is permanently disabled from CMV every ten hours." I am sure these same statistics are true all over the United States.

The CMV virus is a member of the human herpes viruses. It is in the same family as herpes simplex, herpes varicella (chicken pox) and Epstein-Barr (mononucleosis). In 1904, a researcher named Ribbert identified the CMV, but it wasn't until 1920 that it was found to be a virus. This virus was finally isolated in 1956. An infection with CMV is generally asymptomatic, and usually an individual does not know they are infected. Much progress has been made in the last twenty years in understanding this infectious organism, but much more needs to be done.

It is contagious through any body fluids, including saliva, blood, urine, semen, vaginal fluid, or breast milk. Ninety percent of infants appear normal at birth, and 80 percent of infants never have any symptoms. However, being rare is no comfort to that infant and family who are affected.

Congenital cytomegalovirus occurs when an infected mother passes the virus through the placenta. The mother may have no symptoms and not even know she infected. Most congenitally infected infants have no symptoms. Only one out of ten infected infants will have symptoms. These symptoms include: inflammation of the retina, jaundice, enlarged spleen and liver, low birth weight, rash, seizures, and a small head (microcephaly). Psychomotor retardation will be evident shortly after birth.

CMV is the most common cause of non-congenital deafness in children. Infected infants may develop hearing loss or visual impairment as late as two years of age.

Unfortunately, there is no treatment for the virus. It is important that an early diagnosis is made so action can begin immediately to attempt to correct the abnormal development or at least to find ways to compensate.

Since the CMV virus is almost everywhere in the environment, the CDC has recommended the following steps to reduce the spread:

- Wash hands with soap and water after handling diapers or saliva.
- Avoid kissing children on the lips or cheeks.
- Do not share food, drinks, or utensils with young children.
- Pregnant women working in daycare should not work with children under two years of age.

Funding events are always underway to find more support for research in managing this sneaky virus.

Erythroblastosis fetalis, or hemolytic disease of the newborn, is a serious condition that causes jaundice in newborn infants. It occurs in Rh negative pregnant mothers. There is no vaccine to treat this condition but we now have a vaccine which, when given to the pregnant mother, can prevent it from happening. Before the vaccine, however, we had to diagnose the problem at birth and start treatment immediately. This was a disease that could actually be treated, not cured, but treated, to, hopefully, prevent the infant from being damaged.

Mothers who do not have the Rh factor are called Rh negative. If the baby she is carrying has inherited the Rh factor from the father, the infant is Rh positive. If this happens, the mother can develop antibodies against the baby's blood. These antibodies cross the placenta and attack or break apart the infant's red blood cells, resulting in anemia and the release of a pigment called bilirubin. Bilirubin is deposited in the skin and seen as yellow jaundice. The second pregnancy is especially vulnerable to this condition because of previous sensitivity developing in the first pregnancy. In extreme cases, the infant dies before birth or is born with a condition known as hydrops fetalis. This condition is characterized by edema or swelling, heart failure, and anemia. When the amount of bilirubin in the blood exceeds the body's ability to excrete it, it reaches high levels, is deposited in the brain, and causes damage. This brain damage is called kernicterus and is the cause of deafness, spasticity, athetosis, mental retardation, or even death. It was the most common cause of cerebral palsy in children.

In the past, the only treatment we had was to remove this bilirubin and stop the process with a procedure called an exchange transfusion. This was done in the operating room under sterile conditions. A catheter was threaded into the umbilical vein in the naval and a small amount of the newborn's blood containing bilirubin was drawn out (about 10 ml) and discarded. It was then replaced with an equal amount of cross-matched blood from the blood bank that contained no antibodies and no bilirubin. This procedure was carried out over and over and over and over, until all of the infant's blood was completely exchanged and the bilirubin was washed out. This procedure took several hours. If we were lucky, a student nurse or an assistant kept up with the 10 milliliters out – 10 milliliters in monotonous routine until we reached the completion of the exchange. In spite of tired feet, aching legs, and drooping eyes, we were excited to know that we were stopping a death-dealing process, or at least preventing a lifelong condition of spastic cerebral palsy.

A milder form of jaundice can be caused by other conditions. In the late 1950s, an astute nurse noted that babies exposed to sunlight streaming through the nursery window did not become as jaundiced as others. Apparently, the rays of sunlight change the bilirubin to a chemical that is more easily excreted. This observation led to the use of phototherapy to keep the amount of bilirubin from reaching dangerous levels. Apparently, a blue fluorescent light shining on the baby acts the same as sunlight and changes the bilirubin into a different chemical compound that is water-soluble and is then excreted in the urine and the stool. It does not cross into the brain, thus damage to the brain is prevented. This simple observation led to a historic change in treatment of infants, and today, many infants are placed under the lights.

In 1963, a young obstetrician named Vincent Freda (along with John Gorman) developed a substance that would block the antibodies and prevent the jaundice from developing. This substance was made into a vaccine called Rhogam, and it is now a standard treatment for Rh negative pregnant women. Today, very few infants are faced with the dangerous exchange transfusion procedure and pediatric residents are rarely faced with this task.

By treating mothers, many infants can be saved from the life-altering fate of developing cerebral palsy. Like all vaccines, the physician must give the vaccine and the mother must accept it.

CHAPTER ELEVEN

Cerebral Palsy

Robert and Catherine were proud parents of a son, Michael. He was born full term after several episodes of premature labor and rapid fetal heart beats during the last three months of pregnancy. For the first few months of life, he was floppy. Their pediatrician insisted he would "catch up," but Catherine continued to be worried. He was slow to sit, and by nine months of age, his lower extremities felt stiff, making diapering difficult. The diagnosis was cerebral palsy, probably secondary to brain damage before birth.

Cerebral palsy (CP) can be loosely translated to mean "brain paralysis." It is an umbrella classification that covers a large number of problems in children, characterized by disorders of movement, posture, and balance. It is caused by abnormal development or damage in specific locations in the brain. These are the parts that control muscle tone and motor activity. No method has been found to repair the damage. It varies in the way it presents: by the part of the brain affected, by the severity of the damage, and by the quality of the therapy the child receives. Luckily, CP is usually not progressive. But it can get worse by secondary complications such as contractures of joints, seizures, and other medical complications. It is the most common cause of childhood disability.

When children have problems with the motor system, it becomes obvious early in life. Parents place a great emphasis on rolling over, crawling, sitting, and walking. Baby books and videos are usually filled with pictures of that first step. When motor function is delayed, everyone begins to worry. These delays are one of the most common reasons that parents bring children in for an evaluation. Late sitting up, problems rolling over, or not walking at an acceptable age create anxiety in every parent. Abnormal muscle tone, a hand preference before the age of one, and very brisk reflexes are signs to be wary of. Wise parents will not listen to well-meaning neighbors and friends who reassure them with "Just be patient; when he starts you will not be able to catch him." A thorough evaluation by a knowledgeable professional will either reassure the parent that it is, indeed, a normal variation or find the problem and search for answers. Even though CP is usually diagnosed by a careful examination, it is important to be sure that underlying diseases or conditions are causing the symptoms. CT scans, MRIs, or cranial ultrasonography can be helpful in finding the cause, but they are not necessary to make the diagnosis.

Most experts believe that about 80 percent of all CP is caused by prenatal factors. Prematurity, lack of oxygen to the brain, bleeding in the brain, injury during childbirth or in early childhood, extreme jaundice, and genetic factors are the most common causes of the damage. CP needs the efforts of a working team because of the complexity of the condition. In this case, the cause is not as important as defining what the child can and cannot do. When that is determined, a therapeutic program can be developed.

Many children with cerebral palsy have at least good intelligence, although a deficiency in intelligence can occur. Difficulty in communication can give the appearance of mental deficiency. One of my good friends was Clyde Berger, the librarian at the Institute of Logopedics in Wichita, Kansas. He had cerebral palsy caused by jaundice at birth from Rh incompatibility in his mother. His speech was difficult to understand and he walked with canes and braces, but he ran an outstanding library. His wonderful attitude made me forget he had a problem. In 1981, he published a book about his disability. It was called *Grandpa's Boy, and What Became of Him.* It is a deeply moving autobiography about how his grandpa helped him with his struggle to find his place in life.

The management of CP can involve medications. Botulium toxin has been used to relax the spasms of individual muscles; however, it only will last about three to six months. Other medications, when aimed at targeted symptoms, can be helpful. The truly effective treatments are intensive physical therapy, occupational therapy, speech and language therapy, and a good, skilled special education teacher. An experienced orthopedic surgeon can help prevent or correct the contractures and deformities that often develop.

Cerebral palsy is classified in several categories, according to the type of disability. They are: spastic hemiplegia, when one side of the body is affected; spastic diplegia, when both lower extremities are affected; athetoid dyskenesis, when abnormal movements are prominent; and hypotonic, when the child has decreased tone and is floppy. A category called mixed is a frequent finding. There are other classifications that are not used as often. The most important point to remember is that CP is a static condition and usually does not progress in severity.

Robert and Catherine enrolled Michael in physical therapy, speech and language therapy, and had him fitted with braces. He used a wheelchair in pre-school. He was a whiz at computers and used them for his communication. The use of computers and all the advancements in computer science has opened many doors, especially in the world of adaptive communication. I have worked with many children who have learned to use a stylus with their mouth to type out messages. His parents worked with him, and so did his older sister. This positive effort by the whole family was a miracle to watch. An outstanding speech therapist and a knowledgeable special education teacher both invested in Michael. He was able to adjust to his challenge and to find his place in society.

United Cerebral Palsy is a large and successful organization that has been working with great success helping to improve the functioning of thousands of children. In the 1940s, there was little help for children with CP. Many were excluded from schools, and children with all disabilities were treated like second-class citizens. There was a lack of understanding and a fear of the unknown that pervaded society. Parents were often told to place their damaged child in institutions. Parents felt alone and isolated.

In 1948, Leonard Goldenson, president of ABC television, and Jack Hausman, a New York businessman, both had sons with cerebral palsy. With their wives, Isabelle and Ethel, they ran an ad in the *New York Herald Tribune* and asked parents with affected children to join with them in searching for help and ways to improve their children's lives. Hundreds of families responded and that was the beginning of United Cerebral Palsy. It was formally founded in 1949, and is one of the most effective non-profit organizations in the country. This program raises money via telethons and sponsors clinics, treatment programs, and research. They can be extremely helpful to parents, and I have advised all of my parents with a CP child to join and become an active participant.

Michael goes to school in his special wheelchair that has a motor and a number of computerized enhancements. He is well-loved by his teachers and, more importantly, by his classmates.

CHAPTER TWELVE

Muscular Dystrophy

The muscular dystrophies are a group of genetic disorders that result in muscle weakness over time. There is no cure (yet). The condition can become severe, with difficulty breathing and cardiac failure. It is estimated that there are 1 in 5000 to 7000 males between the ages five to twenty-four years with this condition. About 90 percent are in wheelchairs by the age of twenty-four.

Jack's father said he was four years old, but Jack said he was "four and a half." He loved sports and, especially, baseball. Jack was a little underweight and looked like he could use a few more pounds. His father, by contrast, was large, muscular, and had the look of an athlete. He took his son out every day after work to practice ball and had become worried when he noticed Jack seemed to become less coordinated as he grew older. Recently, he had trouble getting up when he fell. The family said maybe he needed more sleep or maybe he needed to eat better or maybe he needed vitamins. All of these maybes were brought to me to find the answer. There was not a good answer.

After a careful evaluation, it was clear that Jack had muscular dystrophy (MD). During the exam, Jack had to use his hands to push on his knees and finally his hips, to get up from the floor. This is called the Gower's sign, and is a classical finding in MD. It is due to muscle weakness in the legs and hips. A muscle biopsy and an elevated blood CPK confirmed the clinical diagnosis. Jack said, "I'll be okay. My dad says I just need to rest more."

Pediatricians are frequently approached by parents when a child is "late" walking or has other motor delays. The average age of diagnosis of muscular dystrophy is five years, yet parents may notice early symptoms at around two and a half years. This delay hinders the onset of early intervention and access to other medical treatments. Parents need access to accurate information as early as possible. Even though neuromuscular diseases are rare, we need to be alert to the symptoms and findings as early as possible.

An early diagnosis alerts the family to obtain genetic counseling and family planning. The CDC and others have developed a web-based tool to assist practitioners to evaluate these children more accurately. The web address is ChildMuscleWeakness.org. The American Academy of Pediatrics advises physicians to look for the "signs of weakness by age." These include:

- Head lag in infants when pulled to sitting position
- A six-month-old who cannot achieve and maintain a sitting position
- A twelve-month-old who cannot rise to stand from the floor and walk and run

Other red flags include irregular movements of the tongue, loss of motor milestones, and a CPK blood level that is three times the normal.

Some of the bravest children I have ever had the pleasure of working with were those with muscular dystrophy. This is a devastating condition, but somehow these kids seem to be able to find joy in life and display it with a smile. As we watch them struggle to stand and take whatever steps are possible, our heart aches to help them. Not a single one has ever asked me to help them. It is amazing to watch how they play games in their wheelchairs and have exciting races with their friends. Often, an older child will become a strong advocate for one of the new kids and the encouragement and support will make the difference between accomplishment and failure.

There are nine types of dystrophy, and Jack had the one called Duchenne. In 1868, a French neurologist named Guillaume Duchenne described thirteen boys with muscle weakness. He pioneered a revolutionary diagnostic test that included taking a small piece of muscle and examining it under the microscope. He carefully described the diagnostic findings indicative of MD. This biopsy is the standard we still use today. He described a specific form of muscular dystrophy that now carries his name. Duchenne MD is the most common type and occurs in 1:3500 male births. The next most common is Beckers MD, which occurs in 1:30,000 births. Other types are even rarer. They all have progressive muscle weakness.

The major cause of MD is an abnormality in the genetic code on the short arm of the X chromosome passed on to the child from the mother. This defect results in the decreased or absent production of the muscle protein called dystropin. This protein is necessary for muscle growth and action. When it is abnormal or absent, the muscles cannot function as they should. Defective dystrophin production causes cellular instability and the leakage of CPK into the blood, resulting in a high level of this enzyme. Eventually, the muscle cell dies and is gradually replaced by fibro-fatty infiltrate, giving the muscle an enlarged and bulky look. On first glance, it appears that the muscle has overgrown, but this is called pseudohypertrophy. It is easily seen in the calf muscle. Spinal deformities and soft tissue contractures usually develop due to poor posture caused by the muscle weaknesses. Sometimes, a wheelchair child will be limited by the developing scoliosis of the spine, causing pressure on the chest and a decrease in the lung capacity. Unfortunately, Duchenne MD is a terminal disease. Most children with MD do not live beyond age thirty, and many die before that age. Death is frequently due to respiratory infections and cardiopulmonary failure.

Jack's parents only knew about muscular dystrophy from the famous telethon that was broadcast every Labor Day on television sponsored by the Muscular Dystrophy Association, with Jerry Lewis as the sponsor and spokesman. This telethon has raised millions of dollars to fund research, clinics, and other efforts to help these children and their families. Jerry, a famous comedian and movie star, became an extremely successful advocate for children until his health forced him to retire. The telethon in 2014 raised over 59.9 million dollars, but was the last year of the telethon. Recently, the MDA joined hands with the Amyotrophic Lateral Sclerosis foundation (ALS) and sponsored the Ice Bucket Challenge, which raised 100 million dollars in 2015.

Research sponsored and funded by the telethon and the National Institute of Health was successful in identifying the defect in the gene responsible for the protein dystrophin. It's not caused by diet, lack of activity, too much activity, toxins, or any of those causes suggested by his grandparents and well-meaning friends. It is a genetic condition that exists on the X chromosome, so it is passed from the mother to her son. Variations exist, leading to various types of MD.

"What do we do?" were the stress-filled words from the father. He was an avid athlete and had envisioned his son following in his footsteps. The majority of these boys do not live past their teen years. Our primary task is to help them achieve the highest quality of life that is possible. Usually their intelligence is adequate, so these children can actively participate in a treatment program. The professionals I have found the most helpful have been occupational therapists and physical therapists. When they accept the responsibility of being the advocate for the child, wonderful things happen. The most remarkable children I have ever seen have been those with dystrophy who maintain an outstanding attitude. Whether it is braces or wheelchairs, nothing seems to get them down.

The medication treatment of MD, so far, has been disappointing. The drug drisapersen was tested in clinical trials in 2012 but failed to show the improvement that was hoped for. In 2015, a new drug, named eteplirsen, developed by Sarepta Therapeutics, has shown encouraging positive results in clinical studies. The FDA is considering its approval for clinical treatment. This drug is designed to work on the underlying cause of the disease by increasing the production of dystrophin. We all continue to hope for success.

Boys with MD experience progressive muscular weakness. Corticosteroids are the only approved drugs we have today that increase muscle strength. The benefits include an increase in the length of time that boys with MD can walk, a reduction in spinal scoliosis, a longer time of adequate breathing, and possible protection against heart problems. However, there are numerous undesirable side effects to steroids.

The National Institute of Neurological Disorders is beginning a clinical research project to determine which steroid gives the best results with the fewest side effects. It will take place in forty-two centers around the world. Any parent interested in this project should contact the National Institute of Health (www.ninds.nih.gov/disorders/clinical_trials).

The 2012 ambassador for the Muscular Dystrophy Association was an eleven-year-old young man from North Carolina named Bryson Foster. He is an avid sports fan, full of wit, and an outgoing speaker. His wheelchair never slows him down and he gives many speeches to raise funds for the research, in hope of finding a cure. The Muscular Dystrophy Association has been an avid and successful advocate for dystrophy since 1950. It was started by a group of adults with dystrophy, their parents, and a physician/scientist. It now sponsors more than 200 clinics across the country and supports more than 300 research projects. Every parent faced with a child with MD should join this successful parent advocacy group.

If we can guide Jack's parents to succeed in helping him live his life to the fullest, in spite of this overwhelming challenge they face, our reward will be the smile on Jack's face.

CHAPTER THIRTEEN

Deaf and Hard of Hearing

When I met Elliot, he was six years old. He was a delightful little boy with numerous freckles on his nose and a quick, enticing smile. He spoke to me with clear, distinct words. He had been found to have a profound congenital hearing loss by the newborn screening test at birth. He was proud of the pretty blue hearing aids that he had worn since he was six weeks old.

It was not easy. The mother said that, when they screened him for hearing as her second newborn, she had no idea the impact that test was going to have on their family. She and Elliott had been discharged from the hospital and were ready to leave. The discharge nurse said, "I need to do a screening test on the baby before you leave. It will only take about fifteen to twenty minutes." The parents did not know what the screening test was all about. They were anxious to leave, but a few more minutes wouldn't hurt.

After over an hour of trying, the tester said, "It's probably nothing, but after many attempts, I can't get this machine to show any response. Don't worry, we'll retest him in two weeks."

The parents weren't worried because they didn't understand what the test was about. However, when they returned for the retest, there still was no response. They were given the test results and told, "Take this to your pediatrician and see what she says."

The pediatrician said, "It may not be anything, but take him to an audiologist or an ENT physician to see if it's serious."

A Child is Waiting

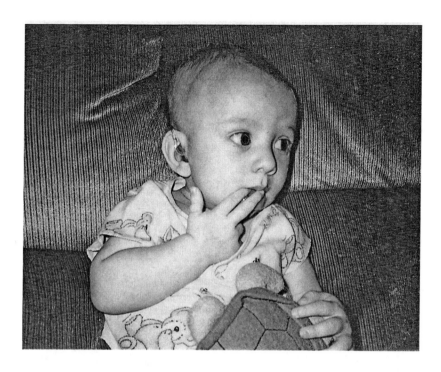

It was! Elliott had profound congenital hearing loss. The cause was unknown. They enrolled him in the Sunshine Cottage for the Deaf, and he was fitted with pretty blue hearing aids and placed in a class for infants. At age six weeks, he was sitting quietly in his car seat wearing his new blue hearing aids.

They turned on the aids for the first time, and his dad said, "Hi, Elliott." Elliott screamed. The shocked parents realized that these were the first words Elliott had ever heard. The parents broke down in tears. When I met him, he was speaking at the same level as all six-year-old hearing children.

Hearing impairment is a threat to the development of language, socialization, and emotional strength. It is also a threat to academic achievement. Early diagnosis and appropriate intervention will improve the outcome. Profound hearing loss is rare but milder loss is commonplace. The word *deaf* is used only when the loss is in the profound range and only a few elements of phonetic speech are heard.

About 50 percent of hearing loss is due to genetic factors. Autosomal recessive inheritance is where both parents carry a recessive gene but have no hearing loss. They pass on the hearing loss genes to the child, resulting in a hearing loss. This is responsible for about 70 percent of congenital loss. About 15 percent of congenital loss is due to an autosomal dominant gene passed on to the child from one parent who may have a hearing loss.

The other 50 percent of hearing loss is due to perinatal, prenatal, or postnatal factors. Non-genetic causes of loss include maternal infections, prematurity, birth injuries, toxins, toxemia, and prenatal lack of oxygen. There are genetic syndromes that can also cause congenital hearing loss, including Down syndrome, Wardenburg syndrome, and Treacher-Collins syndrome.

There are two types of loss after birth and a category of a mixture of these two. Conductive loss is due to a mechanical interference with the sound reaching the cochlea or the nerves to send an impulse to the brain. This type of loss usually will result in a loss that is not as severe and can frequently be repaired. A sensorineural loss is the most serious and is due to a problem with the inner ear or the nerve pathways.

To realize that a child has a hearing loss is not as easy as it should be, as infants and children adapt quickly to the problem and the adjustment can mask the defect. Clapping the hands or slamming a door are not tests of hearing.

Congenital hearing loss is present from birth and usually the entire family, the pediatrician, and everyone around will miss it. When the loss is finally diagnosed, the family will feel guilt, grief, and anger that it had not been detected sooner. When I began to study hearing loss, I was very surprised to find that in almost every baby with a hearing loss at birth, it is missed for several years by everyone. For someone who is not trained, it is extremely difficult to detect a hearing loss in babies, as the common test of clapping your hands, slamming a door, or blowing a whistle and watching the reaction is completely ineffective

After attending a workshop on detecting and treating hearing loss in infants, given by experts from around the country, we realized that newborn infants can be accurately screened for a hearing loss. We also learned that if the loss is detected before six months of age *and is treated*, children will develop language equal to their cognitive abilities by age five. This type of neonatal screening is done by attaching a small electrode to the baby's head. A sound is sent to the baby's ear. The brain will react to the signal and this can be seen on an electronic receiver. If there is no reaction from the baby's brain, a hearing loss is suspected and must be evaluated in much more depth. This simple test can be performed by anyone who is taught how to perform it. In many hospitals, it is done by the person who takes the infant's picture.

Armed with this information, we joined forces with a representative of the Texas State Department of Health and Dr. Therese Finitzo, a knowledgeable, expert audiologist. Together, we confronted the Texas legislature and got a bill passed requiring hearing screening at birth of every baby born in the Texas.

HB 714 was passed by the 76th Texas legislature in 1999, and when signed by Governor George W. Bush, it became Texas law. It mandated that every baby born in Texas would be screened for hearing prior to discharge from the hospital. Insurance companies were required to pay for the screening and it required the state to make treatment available.

This accomplishment took tremendous educational efforts to inform many members of the legislature. We had to overcome the objections of powerful lobbying forces, such as the insurance lobby who felt it would "cost too much," and the Texas hospital lobby who said it would "put a strain on hospitals." It was a great day when the law passed, but more importantly, it was a momentous step forward for the infants born in Texas.

The Texas experience has been replicated all over the country. In Texas, there are at least two babies born every day with a significant congenital hearing loss. This bill has had a dramatic impact on many children, by preventing a hearing loss from becoming a disability. Several states had preceded Texas to screen infants for hearing loss and many have been added since then.

Sometimes we seize the opportunity to be an advocate for children without any idea how successful or how effective it will be. It just seems like the right thing to do.

In 2011, 384,146 infants were born in the state of Texas. Of these newborns, 99.4 percent were screened by the Newborn Hearing Screening Program. As a result, 407 infants were found to have a significant hearing loss. That is 407 infants who were started on treatment as infants. These infants will not have to be in special education programs for the deaf. They will not suffer from speech and language deficits. They will not have to learn signing. These parents will not suffer the pain of a child with a major disability. The state will save millions of dollars by avoiding the need for more special education programs.

The statistics for other states have been just as dramatic.

Prevention and early diagnosis are the keys to success in many problems that interfere with children achieving their right to optimum development. In the past, prenatal exposure to the rubella virus was a common cause of congenital hearing loss, but immunization against the German measles virus has been successful in eliminating this cause. Bacterial meningitis due to H. influenza, another cause, has also been conquered with a vaccine. There are many medications that will cause hearing loss in the prenatal period. Every pregnant mother should carefully check with her physician before taking any medication while pregnant.

Middle ear infections and middle ear effusions will also prevent sound from reaching the nerve centers, resulting in a conductive loss.

Medical therapy of a conductive loss frequently involves the determination of whether a fluid-filled middle ear can be medically cleared and, if not, the question of whether tubes should be placed through the tympanic membrane (ear drum). The use of tympanometry is a simple test to detect if fluid is present. It has certainly helped, especially when the eardrum can't be seen clearly. There is no question that judicial placement of tubes to drain the middle ear can be beneficial in preventing conductive loss.

Parents must teach their children that prolonged exposure to very loud music can damage the conductive mechanism. This is especially true if earphones are used on a constant basis.

If all else fails, early diagnosis and adequate treatment can compensate for the loss, and normal or at least adequate language can result. Many children who are diagnosed early and receive adequate therapy, including aids, can achieve acceptable language skills, but it takes intensive speech and language therapy.

In 2011, those 407 children in Texas who were found to have hearing loss were just like Elliott. Elliot's parents are strong supporters of these children and have volunteered to be their advocates at every opportunity. (They gave me permission to tell their story and to share Elliot with my readers.)

The impact of even minor loss can be a serious impairment on the developing child. We know that by the age of four years, the average child will have a complete knowledge of their native language. This is without any training. Even a partial hearing loss will greatly interfere with this natural development. Deafness alone does not impede intelligence but may cause the child to function at a lower level. Academic achievement will certainly suffer.

To detect hearing loss early requires a physician who is alert to the history of risk factors and willing to administer a simple screening test in their office. A test such as the Early Language Milestone scale (ELM) or the Clinical Linguistic and Auditory Milestone Scale (CLAMS) can be administered easily. The revised Denver Developmental Screening Test has a good language section. The key is the suspicion of a problem and the willingness to pursue that suspicion.

Cochlear implants are being used more frequently, as they have been improved and we have gained more knowledge about their placement. Candidates for implants should be more than twenty-four months old, have sensorineural loss, and have shown no improvement with less invasive therapy. There will have to be a consistent dedication of the family to intensive training and a habilitation program. Perhaps, as the technical

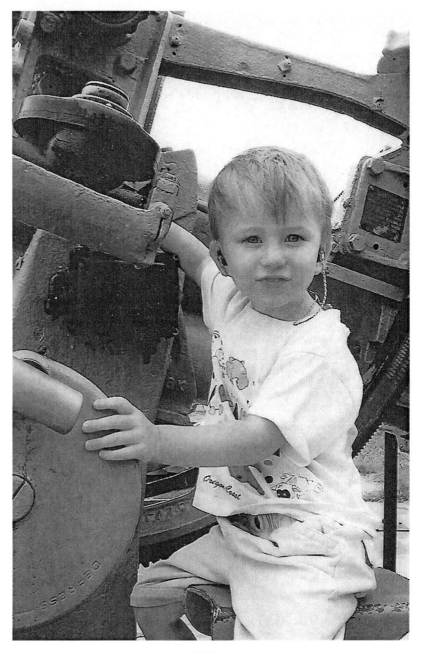

Elliot

aspects of cochlear implants continue to improve, they will be utilized much more often.

The most important and effective therapy for hearing loss is intensive language and speech therapy. This should be started immediately after a diagnosis is made, even without knowing the cause. This therapy will require years. Frequently, behavioral and emotional help will also be required.

The decision on the pros and cons of oral language or sign language is certainly a personal one. A parent should consult experts in the field and find help in making that decision.

The American Society for Deaf Children (ASDC) can be helpful in finding resources, finding support groups and influencing legislation (asdc@deafchildren.org). I strongly advise every parent with a hearing impaired child to join this group.

David Meyers wrote an insightful statement in his book *A Quiet World*:

> Although I wish my hearing were acute, the possibility of severe hearing loss neither frightens nor depresses me. Without deluding myself that other sensitivities will compensate for sensory disability, I am optimistic that I will adapt, that I will develop new sensitivities and that I will drink from other sources of lasting joy.

CHAPTER FOURTEEN
Intellectual Developmental Disability

In 1961, the AAMR introduced the phrase Mental Retardation to replace such inappropriate and demeaning names such as feebleminded, imbecility, or idiocy. It is now time for new, more accurate terminology. In recent years, numerous professional and lay groups have used the term Intellectual Disability (ID). The 2013 issue of the *Diagnostic and Statistical Manual of Mental Disorders (DSM-5)* uses this new terminology. In the 2015 *International Classification of Diseases,* the term will be Intellectual Disability Disorder (IDD). In the US, a federal law (PL-111-256) designated this new term to be used in all federal publications. These terms are interchangeable and represent the critical components of intelligence. They include verbal comprehension, perceptual reasoning, and cognitive efficacy.

The history of how society has confronted children with mental retardation in the past can be a shock to those of us who devote our lives to helping them achieve their rights.

The 1920s was a black period in the history of the United States in the treatment of individuals who deviated from the norm. With the establishment of the American Eugenics Society, a push was made to eliminate the passing on of negative and undesirable traits. As you would expect, these traits were concentrated in the poorer, uneducated, and minority populations. The eugenicists began to drive legislation to prevent "propagation" in these groups. Forced sterilization became the law in thirty states. Over 64,000 people were sterilized. As time went by, the definition of *undesirable* included mentally retarded, but became broader to include those in poverty, the uneducated, the immoral, and the racially different. In 1927, the US Supreme Court ruled it was legal to sterilize Carrie Buck for promiscuity (she had a baby out of wedlock). Justice Oliver Wendell Holmes wrote:

> It is better for all the world, if instead of waiting to execute degenerate offspring for crime, or to let them starve for imbecility, society can prevent those who are manifestly unfit from continuing their kind . . . three generations of imbeciles is enough.

This ruling legitimized the sterilization laws. The state of California had such a robust program that Hitler's Nazi program in Germany used it as a basis for their infamous eugenics program. Following the horrors of Nazi Germany in the 1940s, the eugenics movement began to lose power and was, eventually, completely discredited.

Society continued to treat "those who were different" as if they were a threat. Large institutions were built, some to house over 20,000 individuals, many of them children. Frequently, they were built in the isolated countryside and named deceitful names like Sunnybrook or Willowbrook. This succeeded in removing these unfortunate children and adults as far from society as possible. Doctors told parents to "put them away and forget them." Not only were children who were different confined, but girls who became pregnant, adolescents who acted out, and even individuals who acted strangely were committed. There was no due process. In one institution in Pennsylvania, difficult-to-manage children were kept in four foot by four foot, slatted wooden cages.

The intent was to protect society from these "bad influences," not to protect the child. For many, there was a misunderstanding that a retarded, handicapped, or disabled individual would have an adverse effect on the family and on society. No therapeutic treatment or rehabilitation was available.

In the 1960s, over 156,000 individuals with "mental retardation" and over 550,000 individuals labeled as "mentally ill" were in our institutions in the US, and there were millions more throughout the world.

When the storm of the civil rights social revolution was swirling around us, a quieter but just as meaningful revolution was underway in the world of individuals with disabilities. Supported by President John F. Kennedy and continued by President Lyndon Johnson, the liberating measures and laws that freed those discriminated against by society because of color also freed many individuals who suffered discrimination and neglect because they were different in other ways.

Parents who were trying to keep their handicapped child at home found they were excluded from school. The history of the federal government's attempts to help children with disabilities began in 1857 with the establishment of the Columbia Institution for the Deaf, Dumb, and Blind at Gallaudet University. In 1859, the American Printing House for the Blind was established. Unfortunately, very little was done after those two programs were started. One hundred years later, in 1958, Public Law 85-126 was passed to authorize the training of teachers to work with the mentally retarded.

Finally, sweeping changes were enacted in our educational system when the laws of inclusion were passed in 1963. Started by President Kennedy and finished by President Johnson, Public Law 88-164 declared that no child could be excluded from school, no matter what the cause or the level of their disability. The wording was changed from "the Mentally Retarded" to include children with any handicap. Finally, in 1975, Public Law 94-142, titled "Education for All Handicapped Children," was passed by Congress. It brought together the many amendments and regulations into one sweeping law. The Division of Handicapped Children in the US Office of Education was established. For the first time, children with disabilities had a voice in our government.

The causes of IDD are as variable as there are children with the disorder. Dr. Allan Crocker, in the 1989 *Pediatric Annals*, utilized the following categories:

- Hereditary disorders

- Early alterations of embryonic development
- Pregnancy problems and perinatal morbidity
- Childhood diseases
- Environmental problems and behavioral syndromes

This extensive list emphasizes the variety and limitless causes that can attack the well-being and development of children. It emphasizes the need to carefully evaluate each child. As each child is evaluated, the cause, the current condition, the treatment, and the prognosis can be determined. It is still useful to determine the level of cognitive challenge, utilizing the terms such as mild, moderate, severe, or profound. We must recognize that these terms are mostly for groupings and not for treatment or prognosis. In this day and time, we have moved beyond using specific isolated numbers (although they can be helpful) to categorize and treat a child. It is much more comprehensive and effective to take a child at their functional and developmental level and build a support system to encourage movement to a higher level.

Valid assessment will take into consideration cultural, linguistic, communication, and behavior elements. There may be limits in adaptive skills in the specific community environment where the child lives. There may be weaknesses in some adaptive skills but strengths in others. Each child will require a specific level and type of support, and that level of support guides us in determining the level of the impairment.

We must always keep in mind that support equals improvement. As we begin to build the support system for each individual child, we look at various skill levels. Instruments such as the AAIDD Adaptive Behavioral Scale and the VINELAND Social Maturity Scale are designed to assist in determining the adaptive levels in the following areas: communication, self-care, home living, social skills, community use, self-direction, health and safety, functional academics, leisure, and work. Of course, the age of the child and the skill levels of each area will determine the emphasis of the support system. An example would be an individual who would test at the "impaired" level of communication, but who functions at a "normal" level in fine motor skills.

It is clear that no one person, teacher, therapist, or parent can do everything. There must be a team to build an effective support system. Within the context of the child's native talents, there are certain rights every child must be granted. They are the right to the pursuit of happiness and to the best quality of life possible. It is our goal to find a place in society where the support system will allow the individual to live as independently as possible. This support system will help them enjoy the life they have and assure they reach the highest level their potential will allow.

Perhaps one of the most significant developments in the acceptance of children and adults with intellectual disability was the foundation of the Special Olympics. Eunice Kennedy Shriver, the sister of President John Kennedy, started a day camp in her home for children with disabilities. The year was 1962 and there was no place for these children to play or be accepted. Mrs. Shriver and President Kennedy had an older sister who was born with intellectual disability. She underwent a lobotomy at age twenty-three, which left her permanently incapacitated. President Kennedy established a Panel on Mental Retardation. Mrs. Shriver was a member of that panel and she began to encourage many schools and universities to establish sports programs for the disabled. The Special Olympics grew out of this program in 1968. It is now the largest sports program in the world for individuals with disabilities. There were 4.4 million participants in 170 countries this past year. This program has done more to achieve the acceptance of children and adults with disabilities than any other program in the world. It has given handicapped individuals a place to gain self-confidence and self-esteem.

We must be continually aware of the co-morbidity conditions that may accompany any intellectual disability. It can be physical appearance, defects in organs of special senses, and others. A treatment program of any kind must include these factors. An example would be a child with a hearing loss. This child would show an intellectual deficit in the functional level of communication. Any treatment program must also include improvement in hearing or adjustment to the loss.

It is paramount to avoid the emotional crippling that so often occurs. This can interfere with meaningful improvement. Every effort must be exerted to build self-esteem and personal confidence. Recently, the world's first ultra-accessible family fun park was established in San Antonio, Texas. It is specially constructed so that every child, no matter their disability, can join in and enjoy the entire park. It is called Morgan's Wonderland, and is a place where every child can succeed and help build their self-image and self-confidence. See the chapter on "Parent Power" for more about this.

Whether it is called intellectual disability, intellectual developmental disability, cognitively impaired, or mental retardation, it is an incurable condition. It brings out a plethora of emotions in everyone. For the professional who is working with the child, these emotions can result in strength and resolve in an unrelenting search for answers to achieve positive results. Remember, if a child with limitations can be supported to utilize 80 percent of their limited abilities, they may equal a person with unlimited abilities who uses only 10 percent of theirs.

CHAPTER FIFTEEN

Autism

"Why is he like this?" the mother asked in an angry, fear filled voice. "Is he autistic? Can you do anything to help? How did this happen?" Her thirty-month-old son was pulling on his mother's restraining hand and repeating a phrase over and over in a soft voice.

"Click-clack, click-clack, click-clack."

He was a handsome lad with fair skin, deep blue eyes, long curved eyelashes, and a somewhat large head covered with locks of blond hair. He had the build of a small tank and appeared extremely healthy.

His parents were distraught, devastated, angry, and full of guilt.

The worry lines on their faces seemed as if they had been there forever. Their only child had just faded away and now seemed to be in another world.

"I want my baby back," the mom sobbed through her tears.

The father's pain and grief were so deep his voice was a low croak and he could hardly speak. "I knew we should have never given him that MMR shot. Could it be due to the drugs I used in college? Maybe God is punishing us for things we did. What happened? What can we do?"

They brought a picture album filled with early pictures of an active baby, full of life. Each picture clearly showed a bright-eyed infant, obviously full of curiosity and interested in his surroundings. At his first birthday party, they dressed him in a cowboy suit with cowboy boots and a hat. They said he seemed unusually quiet and a little withdrawn. It seemed to get worse, and by sixteen months, he had lost some of the language he'd previously mastered. He could no longer say "mama" or "dada," and his social and emotional development lagged behind his peers. By two years, he had ceased to interact with other children. He was repeating words said to him over and over, like an echo. He held onto a toy wheel and spun it constantly in front of his eyes. When he became frustrated, he screamed and flapped his hands. As the parents and I talked, he wandered aimlessly around the room, never making eye contact with me or with his parents. I deeply felt the pain of these loving parents. Their fears were correct.

Their child was autistic.

He had almost all the symptoms and findings of autism. Most children with autism have a variety and degree of symptoms and an even more variety of findings. Each child is different.

This is one of those conditions where (at this date), the cause is not absolutely known and there is no known cure. An incurable condition represents the most painful diagnosis for any physician to make and the most devastating for all family members. Unfortunately, there are many conditions that are incurable in children. Multiple sclerosis, rheumatoid arthritis, influenza, mental retardation, and several forms of cancer are just a few examples. Perhaps the most representative of an incurable condition that we face today is autism.

By definition, autism is a complex neuro-developmental disorder that results in problems in communication, social interaction, and stereotypical behaviors. It is accompanied by abnormalities in cognitive functioning, learning, attention, and sensory processing. Some of the associated symptoms are extremely disabling, such as aggression and self-injurious behaviors.

Every child with autism does not have every symptom or finding. There is a great deal of variation and degree.

Autism was first described by Eugene Bleuler, an Austrian psychiatrist and physician. In 1911, he published his findings and first used the word *autism*, which he took from the Greek *autos* (self). His theory was that autism was a form of childhood schizophrenia. This theory was altered in 1940s by Leo Kanner, an Austrian psychiatrist, and Hans Asperger, an Austrian scientist and pediatrician. Today, we recognize that there is a spectrum of autism disorders that vary in presentation and in severity.

As of this date, there is no medical test or laboratory evaluation that can be given to make the diagnosis. Instead, the diagnosis depends on the determination of whether a group of symptoms exists, based on parental reports, clinical judgment, and observation of behavioral symptoms. The Autism Diagnostic Observation Schedule (ADOS) was developed by autism expert Dr. Catherine Lord, who is the head of the new Center for Autism and the Developing Brain at New York Presbyterian hospital. It is the gold standard for diagnosing autism spectrum disorders or ruling them out. It can be quickly and reliably administered and has a sensitivity rating of 95 percent, which means the test will yield a correct diagnosis 95 percent of the time.

An additional test developed by Dr. Lord is the Autism Diagnostic Interview (ADI-R). This test gathers information from interviewing the parents. Together, these two tests yield the most accurate assessment of autism spectrum disorders available. Both tests can be used in children from eighteen months and through adolescence and into adulthood. They have also proven to be useful in accurately assessing treatment progress, especially in research programs. It is important that the individual utilizing these tests be trained in the administration of the tests to obtain the best and most accurate results.

Recently, Dr. Samago-Sprouse at George Washington University reported that in nine- to twelve-month-old infants, a head circumference at or above the 75 percentile or at least 10 percent larger than the length of infants and who did not pass the "head tilting reflex" were at risk to develop autism. This finding will need to be verified by other researchers, but may possibly be an aid in early diagnosis.

At this time, the cause of autism has not been proven. The most recent research has shown that there is a genetic component to the cause. If one of identical twins is diagnosed with autism, there is an 80 to 90 percent chance the other twin will be diagnosed also. In fraternal twins, that percent drops to 3 to 10 percent. The CDC reports that the incidence of autism diagnosis is 1:42 for boys and 1:89 for girls. Some question these numbers and believe that the broadening of the definition, the need to have a diagnosis, the need to obtain treatment in the school system, and other factors have caused an over-diagnosis. That is not important to the child who needs help.

There are many theories, with many possible causes being blamed, and there are an unlimited number of guesses. Multiple research projects are underway searching for answers and they are promising and exciting. The range of types of autism, the complexity of the condition, and given that no two autistic children are alike, make finding a single cause very doubtful. We know that altered genetics play a major role, as a number of genes in these children have been found to be flawed. We now know that ASD is extremely heritable, but the exact common genetic cause remains out of our reach. Whether these genetic variations make the child more susceptible to extraneous factors or whether they play a direct role in causing autistic development has not been shown.

We now know that vaccines **do not** cause autism. A significant number of studies have definitely proven this. So that theory can now be discarded.

When genotyping large numbers utilizing a new test called *copy number variations* (CNV), it was found that the defects tend to cluster in genes controlling biologic pathways in neurotransmission. This opens the door to new research that may bring us closer to solving the etiologic puzzle.

In April 2013, Dr. Galan, from Case Western Reserve, reported the use of a new procedure called magnetoencephlography (MEG) in studying autistic children. This test measures functional connectivity from one region of the brain to another. He reported a 94 percent accuracy rate in diagnosing autistic children. This research was on a small sample and needs to be verified, but it is a good example of current research.

Without proven knowledge as to the cause of a condition, it is extremely difficult to disprove a suspected cause. It is difficult to take away a theory if there is nothing to replace it. It takes unwavering faith and trust to accept ideas that are contrary to what parents hope to be true. It is virtually impossible for loving, caring parents to accept the fact that their child has an incurable condition without knowing the cause. Parents and other family members are susceptible to trying anything, no matter how much it will cost or even if it is potentially dangerous. This is certainly understandable if there is a glimmer of hope, but they can be preyed upon by unscrupulous persons offering "cures" that are not real and are unfounded in facts.

"Do you know about those shark tooth injections we can get south of the border?" "We heard of a doctor giving intravenous chelation treatment for $6000 per treatment." "We heard we could help our son by soaking him in a tub full of Epson salts."

Day after day, new and untried treatments are touted, and they are all touted on the Internet. There seems to be as many treatments as there are guesses as to the cause. These therapies give false hope to desperate parents and frequently interfere with their obtaining any valid therapy.

As with many conditions, there are valid treatments for autism that target the symptoms. These treatments can be effective in relieving some of the problems. Physical and occupational therapy, speech therapy, intensive behavioral therapy, dietary manipulations, and special education have been shown to help. They are expensive, difficult to implement, and require a dedication to many long hours of work, but they are worth the effort. Intensive individual special education by a teacher who is familiar with autism or similar disorders is crucial. This program should be undertaken no matter what other treatments are tried. There is no treatment that targets the core symptoms. This is the goal, dream, and prayer of every parent, every physician, every researcher and every teacher.

Medication therapy must be directed toward the specific symptoms that are interfering with developmental progress. Some of the psychotropic medications have been shown to alleviate aggression or self-abuse, antisocial behavior, or irritability. Medications should be targeted for specific behaviors. Autistic children have been shown to be overly sensitive to medications and should be carefully monitored for side effects.

Our difficult task is to help parents choose those valid treatments and not spend their resources and emotional energy on unproven, potentially dangerous, or deceptive ventures.

Parent groups have been shown to be a powerful force to accomplish miracles. They can influence legislation, raise funds, and stimulate research toward finding the answers so desperately desired. We saw this happen to fantastic fruition with the March of Dimes and the conquering of polio. They can stimulate physicians and researchers to listen and act. They can influence the legislature to allocate more funds for research. However, in their desperation, they can also be misdirected and misguided, and thus end up utilizing that same influence to bring on disaster.

Without knowing the cause, it is extremely difficult to be sure of treatment. We are then faced with analyzing the child, identifying the deficits and problems, and initiating a treatment plan to address the specific needs of the individual child. This can be done without knowing the exact cause. With the support and stimulus of parents, more and more money has been allocated toward research in finding the cause and developing effective treatments. In the meantime, teachers and other school professionals will continue to identify the needs and work hard to help these children achieve as good a life as possible.

There are several parent groups that are active not only in the US but across the world. Every parent of an autistic child should participate in at least one of these groups. It will help them keep up with the newest research and provide them with access to other parents faced with similar problems. Always keep in mind that each child is his/her own individual self and what works for one child may not help another. In fact, it might make it worse. All these organizations raise funds to support research, which is the hope of all.

A new study reported in the journal *Cell* in July 2015 gives new hope. To understand the etiology of autism, the researchers grew miniature one cell brains from stem cells taken from autistic children. These cells revealed a genetic mutation resulting in an increase in an inhibitory enzyme causing interference with neurotransmission. Maybe, just maybe, they have found the cause of autism. Could a cure be possible?

CHAPTER SIXTEEN

Diabetes

When she was told she had diabetes, the young lady sitting on the exam table looked at me with blazing eyes filled with anger, fear, and blame. She said, "It's my mother's fault for feeding me so much sugar. I told her she doesn't care what happens to me. My grandmother has diabetes, and she gave it to me." She even blamed me for finding it.

An adolescent doesn't usually like to go to the doctor, and this fourteen-year-old girl was no exception. She was an attractive child except for acne on her cheeks and forehead and the pout and scowl on her face. Her dress was clean and neat, although there was a feeling of neglect in her appearance. It was clear from observation that this child was overweight, with a waist measurement much more than her hips, a telltale sign of diabetes

Her mother recited her symptoms as if she had read the textbook. "High volume urine output, frequent urination, excessive thirst, and hungry all the time, with excessive weight gain this past year."

On exam, the child also had elevated blood pressure and a history of persistent sleep apnea. The grandmother, who was also overweight, had resisted bringing her granddaughter to the doctor. She said she didn't think anything was wrong except, "She doesn't eat right."

A child with diabetes represents the most fragile and vulnerable child in the medical world. It is not something that can be readily seen and pointed to as evidence of a problem. Serious complications slowly present over a period of time. These complications are made worse by poor care and poor control. Blindness, kidney failure, foot ulcers, high blood pressure, obesity, and poor circulation are a few problems that can make life miserable. These children are in great need of an advocate who has a complete understanding of the disease, especially the emotional turmoil that invariably is present.

The only way to help this adolescent is to diffuse her anger and alleviate her fear. *Maybe* it could be accomplished with education. *Maybe*, if she had all the facts and understood about her condition, the anger would subside and she would accept treatment. *Maybe*, if she knew the results of good treatment and knew that her whole world could be improved, she would become cooperative. *Maybe*, if she could trust someone, she could listen to what had to be said. These are big maybes, but worth pursuing.

Even though it would be a teenager's dream to just receive a few pills to make all her troubles go away, that would never be enough to improve her diabetes, her weight, her elevated blood pressure, or her view of life. It was going to take a total lifestyle change to accomplish these miracles.

Starting with the basics and keeping it as simple as possible, we explained to her that almost all the foods we eat—such as bread, potatoes, pasta, rice, milk, and fruit—are converted by the body to sugar. That sugar is stored in the cells, mostly in fat. It is the fuel the body burns for energy. The Beta cells in the pancreas produce a hormone, called insulin, which moves the sugar into the cells. Most of this enzyme action occurs in the muscles, the liver, and in fat. In 1959, it was discovered that there were two types of diabetes. Type I diabetes is called insulin dependent diabetes because the body does not produce enough insulin. The body attacks the pancreas with antibodies and the damaged pancreas does not produce enough insulin. This is an autoimmune condition. Type II diabetes is called insulin resistant diabetes. For a poorly understood reason, the body develops a resistance to insulin. In either case, ingested sugar cannot move into the cells because there is not enough functional insulin. As the body takes in higher and higher amounts of food, especially carbohydrates, the body tries to make more and more insulin. At that point, the body either can't make enough or is resistant to the insulin that is made. When this happens, the sugar is elevated in the bloodstream. This is called hyperglycemia and that's when all the symptoms start to appear.

We don't completely understand why this resistance to insulin develops in type II diabetes. However, there is a direct relationship between obesity, a decrease in physical activity, family genetics, and the onset of diabetes. From 1990 to 1998, the CDC reported an increase of over 33 percent in the diagnosis of type II diabetes in children in the United States. Each day more children are being diagnosed with type II diabetes, now reaching more than 7 percent of the population. It is estimated that only about 14.6 million of those cases have been diagnosed. One out of every ten US healthcare dollars is spent on diabetes.

This teenager needs to understand that she is not alone, as there are many children struggling with this life-threatening problem. A major epidemic is upon society—one with dire health, financial, and life consequences. Medical complications such as cardiovascular problems, high blood pressure, atherosclerosis, blindness, foot ulcers, and neurological problems can occur in both types of diabetes. Probably the most serious complications in diabetes is ketoacidosis. When the body cannot utilize the ingested sugar due to lack of insulin, the body burns fat to get the required sugar for energy. When fat is burned, acids called ketones are released. As these toxic acid levels increase, the symptoms include excessive thirst, nausea and vomiting, abdominal pain, weakness and fatigue, shortness of breath, fruit-scented breath, and mental confusion. If untreated, it can be fatal or lead to brain damage. Diabetic ketoacidosis can be brought on by illness, fever, stress, emotional trauma, surgery, or poor insulin therapy.

If you report the symptoms of diabetes in a child, including increased thirst, hunger, increased urination, fatigue, and occasionally blurred vision, your doctor will conduct simple tests. A fasting blood sugar level greater than 126, a blood sugar level of greater than 200 after an ingestion of a glucose meal, or a random blood sugar level greater than 200 indicate the diagnosis. The measurement of Hemoglobin A1c is a good method, not only as part of the diagnostic workup but for following the results of treatment. Hemoglobin A1C is the measurement of the blood sugar level for the past three months. A level of 5.7 percent and below indicates no diabetes or in good control. A level of 5.7 to 6.4 percent indicates pre-diabetes or adequate control. A level above 6.5 percent indicates diabetes in poor control. It is important to keep this level below 6.5.

Diabetes is not a new condition. As early as 1500 BC, Egyptian records described it in their writings. Later, in the eleventh century AD, *mellitus*, the Latin word for honey, was added to the word *diabetes* and the disease became known as diabetes mellitus. This was done because the "water tasters" who tasted the urine of those suspected of having diabetes found it to be sweet. Since insulin is produced in the pancreas, an early treatment was to feed patients with ground up pancreas from pigs or cows. I am sure many patients gagged and vomited from this disgusting stuff. It was a complete failure.

In 1921, a young Canadian physician named Dr. Frederick Banting worked in a lab in London, Ontario. He was joined by a medical student named Charles Best. They developed a method to extract insulin from the pancreas. In 1922, they injected a young boy who was diabetic with insulin and saved his life. They had found that if insulin was injected into diabetic patients, their blood sugar level came down. This was the first successful treatment of a human being. Dr. Banting received the Nobel Prize for Medicine in 1923.

Unfortunately, many individuals had severe reactions to the insulin extract from pigs. In 1978, an exciting new method was used to produce insulin. The human DNA gene for insulin was inserted into bacteria and this caused the bacteria to produce human insulin. It is called *recombinant DNA insulin* and the treatment of diabetes was changed forever. Finally, effective and available treatment became available for everyone with type I diabetes.

Insulin can be received by injection, insulin pens, jet injectors, or by insulin pump. Unfortunately, no insulin has been developed to take by mouth.

Treatment of type II diabetes is simple but difficult to follow carefully. Insulin is used infrequently in type II diabetes. Learning the symptoms of low and high blood sugar levels will lead to managing the blood sugar levels. Diet and weight control are essential to good control. Regular and consistent physical activity will lower blood sugar levels, burn extra calories, improve blood pressure, improve blood flow, and increase energy level. There are many medications that can be given if the other methods do not completely control the sugar levels. A physician will determine which medication is best for each child. Insulin is rarely utilized in type II diabetes. Preventing complications is an absolute must. Good foot care and smoking cessation (this includes secondhand smoke) are absolutely necessary. Treatment of type I diabetes is to replace the insulin that is not being produced by the body. At this time, insulin can only be given by injection.

The onset of type II can be delayed and sometimes even prevented with major lifestyle changes. When muscles are improved with exercise, the intake of fat and carbohydrates reduced, and body weight reduced, the body can reach a balance, often eliminating the need for diabetic treatment.

These words sound simple, but to actually achieve these results is extremely difficult. If this angry adolescent, her mother, her grandmother, her teacher, her coach, and every other adult in her life can work with the professional diabetic treatment team, they can help her overcome this life-threatening challenge. There is no "penicillin" for diabetes. Anti-diabetic pills can help control the sugar level in type II, but the disease is still there. The pills are not a cure. A total lifestyle change for the whole family is the only true answer. This means an increase in physical activity, a decrease in body weight, and a change in diet. These three changes are extremely difficult, but they are certainly possible. If she and her family can accept this challenge, it will save not only her life, but the lives of her children and perhaps those of future generations.

The real question for her parents and all the adults in her life remains: we know she is "worth it," but are she and her family willing to pay the price to change her lifestyle and the lifestyles of all those around her? If the entire family can change, the chances of success increase exponentially. Diabetes is a lifelong disease and there is no cure, but a healthy, productive lifestyle can be achieved if the disease is accepted and managed.

CHAPTER SEVENTEEN

Overweight and Obesity

Freddy Jr. was a beautiful little boy sitting quietly on his mother's lap. His birthday was two days ago and he had just turned three. The mother was worried because he was less active than the other kids in daycare. His physical exam was completely normal except for his weight. He was 37.5 inches tall (50th percentile) and his weight was 38.5 pounds (95th percentile). On the CDC calculator, his BMI calculated at 19.2, which placed him at the obese level. His mother said "I keep hoping it is just baby fat and he will lose it soon."

This little child is already headed for trouble. Unless action is taken soon, his risk for dire medical, social, and psychological consequences are greatly increased. These predictions are not just guesses but are based on thousands of studies proving to everyone that obesity as a child will not only result in pain and suffering but will shorten life. There is a 70 percent chance that he will be an overweight adult.

The CDC reports that childhood obesity has more than doubled in the past thirty years. The number of obese six- to eleven-year-olds has increased from 7 percent in 1980 to 18 percent in 2012. The number of obese adolescents has increased to 21 percent. *Overweight* means an excess weight from all body elements, including muscle, bone, fat, and water. *Obesity* means an excess of fat. During my training, nutrition, including obesity, was not even discussed. There was certainly no training on how to manage it. As with diabetes, many conditions contribute to the epidemic, including genetic, biological, emotional, and environmental factors. However, there is one basic fact and it is very simple. If you take in more calories than you burn, you become first overweight, then obese.

There is no need to make it more complicated than that. How can you tell how many calories you burn? It is simple! Weigh on a morning upon awakening and weigh two weeks later at the same time. If you weigh the same, then you are burning close to the same amount of calories that you have ingested. This is true no matter the source of calories. By the way, in spite of what friends tell you, less than 2 percent of overweight individuals have an endocrine problem.

If you want to GAIN weight, take in more calories or burn less calories.

A calorie is a unit of energy, supplied by whatever you take into your body. A calorie is a calorie, no matter the source. Carbohydrates, fat, protein, and sugar all contain calories. You must reduce your calorie intake by 3500 calories to lose ONE pound. If your energy burn stays the same and you reduce your intake by only 100 calories a day, you will lose ONE pound in thirty-five days.

This alarming increase in obesity in our world has dire consequences for the future of our kids and for society. Excessive weight gain leads to high blood pressure, resulting in cardiovascular disease. Sleep apnea and poor sleep patterns are seen in many overweight children. This results in fatigue, lack of energy, and poor school progress. Orthopedic problems are also a common consequence of obesity, especially problems with hips and knees. A significant study revealed an increased risk for back disease in overweight and obese kids. Obesity slows down the healing of disk injuries, including after surgery and physical therapy.

The mental and social anguish suffered by overweight children can be devastating to lifetime success. It breaks my heart when I see a group of children playing and one overweight child is sitting on the side because he can't keep up with the other kids and is teased relentlessly. Remember, it has been shown that overweight children have a 70 percent chance of becoming overweight adults. These adults are more at risk to develop heart disease, type II diabetes, stroke, several types of cancer, and osteoarthritis. Not only is this a tragedy for the obese adult but a burden and drain on society.

Remember, if you take in more calories than you burn, you get fat.

A 2007 study revealed that, nationwide, over 18 percent of African-Americans, 14 percent of Hispanic children, and 11 percent of Caucasian children are significantly overweight. It has steadily climbed to higher levels since that time. They are not "just chubby," but obese. I strongly suspect that these statistics are understated. The percentage is much higher in many specific areas of our country and in the world.

The increasing incidence of obesity, and the often resulting diabetes, represents a worldwide health catastrophe happening before our eyes. It is easy for a physician to diagnose these chronic conditions, but no physician can cure them. The treatment must be the responsibility of every adult in the child's life. Parents, grandparents, teachers, coaches, physicians, and everyone else in the community of the child must accept the responsibility. It is the child's future, but any adult who leaves the changes that must occur to someone else contributes to the problem. We must find a way to mobilize all resources and to guide the family in utilizing them. To do anything less is not acceptable.

The behavior of children toward a healthy lifestyle is influenced by a variety of factors, including families, communities, schools, day care centers, medical care providers, government agencies, faith based institutions, the media, food and beverage industries, and the entertainment industry. It would be impossible to point out one and say, "You are the guilty one." We can, however, ask each of these sectors of society to take an active role in treating and preventing this life threatening development affecting our children. Each one could and should analyze their role in contributing to the problem. They, then, could make significant changes.

The parents are the key. This is a parenting problem, and failure represents parenting failure. That old adage "we are what we eat" has never been more true than today. It has been pointed out that much obesity begins in the infant–toddler age. The pediatrician, the family physician, and the preschool teacher or the day care worker are usually the only professionals who have contact with the child prior to school. They must accept the responsibility of intervening in the family when the overweight condition first begins to appear. These professionals should weigh and measure each child frequently, and chart them on the height–weight graph and calculate the basal metabolic index.

Yes, this should be done by every daycare facility. Parents should be given this graph to take home, to follow and understand where their child lands on the chart. The parents must be counseled on the child's condition. Parents must insist that this be done and must accept the responsibility to correct unacceptable conditions. The pediatrician or the family physician can be the leading influence in mobilizing all the resources available, but so can teachers, coaches, and other influential adults. To do anything less is physician failure and parent failure.

When a child is overweight and becomes an obese adult, we must consider that a total community failure.

Genetics may dictate whether the gene for diabetes, arthritis, obesity, or other chronic condition is present, but a positive attitude and lifestyle changes can keep these conditions from ruining a life.

An accurate food diary and a physical activity diary will surprise everyone. Here are a few web sites to help:

- www.cdc.gov/healthyweight/calories/index.html
- www.cdc.gov/healthyweight/pdf/physicalactivitydiary.htm
- www.blubberbuster.com/height_weight.html
- nccd.cdc.gov/dnpa (body mass index calculator)

With this information, shared with everyone in the child's community, a program can be started. This program should include a careful history of eating patterns, weekly goal setting, and setting up a contract, praise, continual re-assessment, and home environmental controls. The enthusiasm of all involved will motivate the child to join the exciting effort. Can you, the teacher, take on this extra effort? Can you, the parent, take on this extra effort? How about the coach, the minister, rabbi, or priest? Where are Grandma and Grandpa, the aunts and uncles? It is time for pressure on the food and beverage industries. Those movie stars, TV stars, writers, and producers must be influenced to enroll in the war. Let's not forget the strong influence of the hero of our sports teams.

There must be an all-out effort to realize the goal of saving our kids.

CHAPTER EIGHTEEN
Visual Impairment and Blindness

Elizabeth was the first-born of a NBICU nurse. Because of her job with premature infants, this mother was extremely sensitive to her new little girl's development. She had seen many infants develop problems and was determined to detect any deviation from "normal" in her little girl. She was surprised and shocked when she saw the pictures of Elizabeth's first birthday party. The left eye did not have a red reflex and appeared white. The right eye had a red reflex. She immediately took her to her pediatrician, who referred her to an ophthalmologist. This beautiful little one-year-old had a retinoblastoma. This is a rare cancer of the retina, the innermost lining in the back of eye that receives light and images and sends it to the brain. She received radiation therapy and suffered all the side effects. It appears that she has completely recovered, even though the vision in that left eye will never be normal. It was discovered early enough that enucleation (removal) of the eyeball was not needed.

About 250 children are diagnosed with retinoblastoma in the US every year. In 20+ percent of them, it occurs in both eyes. Unfortunately, some are not diagnosed early enough and the tumor is in both eyes or it is too late for successful treatment.

Early diagnosis of visual problems is crucial for treatment of any eye problem to be successful. In the first three months of life, it is normal for the infant's eyes to be "crossed" or even to focus past your face, but if this persists past three months, have it checked. There are certain signs that should alert you to visual problems. They are:

- The eyes don't move normally. One moves and the other doesn't, or one turns and stays that way.
- After one month, lights, mobiles, etc. don't catch the infant's attention.
- One eye doesn't open.
- One or both eyes look cloudy.
- Your baby squints or rubs his eyes.

Vision can be checked in an infant, so don't let anyone tell you that your baby is too young to be evaluated.

Blindness or severe visual impairment has been an enigma for society since primitive times. Mankind has always been afraid of darkness. The early Egyptians were the first civilization to even take an interest in disabilities. Blind individuals were mostly found in the arts or in music and were depicted on wall paintings. Many harpists were blind. It was not until the mid-1700s that "asylums" to train (not educate) the blind began to appear.

In 1821, Louis Braille heard of a communication system used by the army to send information at night. It was called "night writing" and consisted of pinpricks on heavy paper. Braille, who was blind, said, "We do not need pity, nor do we need to be reminded that we are vulnerable. We must be treated as equals and communication is the way this can be brought about." At the age of fifteen, he developed and published the first set of the Braille alphabet. After several revisions, his Braille method was accepted as the national standard for tactile reading in 1918. The American Printing House for the Blind, which was established in 1858, reports that, in 2014, it had 60,393 members. Over 5,147 children received Braille readers. It also reported that 17,647 children received large print readers, 5,529 received auditory readers, 21,042 were non-readers, and 11,028 were pre-readers.

The American Foundation for the Blind was established in 1921 and the National Federation of the Blind was established in 1940. The NFB is the largest organization of its kind in the US and is available to help any family with visual impairment. The

AFB states that the real problem of blindness is not the loss of eyesight itself, but "is found in the wide range of public misunderstandings, misconceptions, and superstitions about blindness held by the sighted as well as the blind."

In 1975, Congress passed the Individuals with Disabilities Act (IDEA) and this has led to the placement of blind students in public schools. Of course, much more needs to be done to make this successful, but it is slowly improving. In 2006, the NFB convinced Congress to mint a commemorative coin to honor Louis Braille on his 200th birthday. The NFB will receive approximately four million dollars from the coin sales to use for Braille projects.

The American Community Survey in 2012 reported the prevalence of visual impairment to involve over 659,700 children age four to twenty years. This is a surprising number and indicates that the prevalence of visually impaired children is a significant educational challenge for our public schools.

The definition of blindness varies according to the various organizations. The "legal blind" definition is that central visual acuity must be 20/200 or less with the best possible correction or that the visual fields must be 20 degrees or less. The National Federation of the blind uses a more reasonable, broader definition. They state that a person should consider themselves blind if their sight is bad enough, even with corrective lenses, that they must use alternative methods to engage in the activities a person with normal vision would do using their eyes. There are no acceptable definitions for visually impaired, low vision, or vision loss. Total blindness means the inability to discern light.

If an infant is born blind or with a severe vision loss, it is crucial to find the cause immediately. The most common cause today is retinopathy of prematurity. The improvement in survival of premature infants has increased this treatable abnormality. It usually occurs in infants born before 31 weeks of pregnancy. It is associated with the use of high concentrations of oxygen therapy. There is a significant abundance of blood vessels in the retina interfering with vision. Most of these infants will require no treatment, but infants with more severe involvement will need surgical treatment by laser therapy. It is advisable for every premature infant who has received oxygen therapy to have a retinal exam, preferably by a retinal specialist. *Prevention* of loss is so much better than *treatment* of loss.

The incidence of congenital cataracts has greatly decreased due to the vaccine that has reduced the number of rubella (German measles) cases. Rubella was the most common cause of cataracts in the past. Some infections, such as cytomegalovirus will result in visual loss. In about 20 percent of infants with reduced vision, the cause will be in the central nervous system and the brain favors the other eye. This can result in amblyopia. Brain damage from any cause can result in neurological visual impairment. In this case, the eyes are normal but the receiving area of the brain does not interpret the incoming visual information.

Some of the common conditions are milder, but if untreated can cause disaster. A "lazy eye" is the result of the vision in one eye being reduced and the muscle balance between eyes is disturbed. If uncorrected, the affected eye will lose its viability, sometimes permanently. This is called amblyopia. Strabismus is the misalignment of the eyes and will result in amblyopia if untreated. Visual screening in the preschool years will detect these problems so they can be corrected. Nearsightedness, farsightedness, and astigmatism are common but easily treated if found and corrected.

Gogate, Gilbert, and Zin, in an excellent review in the *Middle Eastern African Journal of Ophthalmology* point out the importance of early detection of visual loss. They state that blindness and visual impairment in infants is not difficult to detect and diagnose. With proper care, most of these infants can be helped and the formation of amblyopia can be prevented. Even if the physician may not be able to help medically or surgically, optical aids and rehabilitation can help these children reach their full potential.

One cannot write about vision problems without including Helen Keller. She was born on June 27, 1880, as a physically healthy infant. At the age of nineteen months, she contracted a

Vernon L. James, MD

severe illness thought to be scarlet fever. When she recovered, she had lost her hearing and her sight and became mute. Five years later, on the advice of Alexander Graham Bell, the parents obtained a teacher, Anne Mansfield, who taught her to read with Braille and to use the hand signals of the deaf-mute. She went on to receive a college education. During her junior year at Radcliffe College, she published her first book, *The Story of My Life*. It is still in print, in over fifty languages.

Her impact as an educator, organizer, and fundraiser was enormous. Keller and Sullivan were the subject of a play by William Gibson named *The Miracle Worker*. It opened on Broadway in 1959 and as a motion picture in 1962. She was one of the co-founders of the ACLU. Her courage, intelligence, and dedication combined to make her a symbol of the triumph of the human spirit. In 1924, Helen called upon the Lions Club to become the Knights of the Blind.

Responding to that challenge, the Lions International established save vision programs and have helped millions of visually impaired individuals improve their lives. Their most recent endeavor, Sight First, was conceived in 1988 as a global program and is just getting underway. Julie Foeman, an editor of *IN FOCUS* magazine, writes in the *Archives of Ophthalmology* that the blind prevention strategies adopted by Lions International are:

- To develop and/or strengthen the primary care infrastructure by building hospitals, clinics, and mobile eye care clinics
- To develop manpower and managerial skills by providing ophthalmologists, eye care auxiliaries, and surgical assistants
- To promote community mobilization
- To further operations research

The Lions have pledged $100 million to accomplish these lofty goals. The first eight projects are now underway.

Today, most blind students attend public schools aided by regular teachers of academics and a team of specialized helpers.

Blind children especially need help and training in understanding spatial concepts and in self-care. Since only about 10 percent of visually impaired children are legally blind and have no usable vision, all efforts should be made to teach those who have any vision at all how to use what they have. A combination of training targeted to the individual needs of each child will result in blind and visually impaired students capable of dealing with and living in the world independently.

In the United States, there are several organizations available to help parents with a visually impaired child. Every parent should contact these organizations and enroll. Almost all of their services are free.

- The National Federation of the Blind
- The American Printing House for the Blind
- The American Action Fund for Blind Children
- The American Foundation for the Blind,
- Many government agencies
- Your local Lions Club

CHAPTER NINETEEN

Problems of Attention, Learning Differences

When Thomas came to the office, the entire staff would become upset. He was the wildest, most uncontrollable little five-year-old we had ever seen. He had been expelled from three pre-school programs and was now giving his kindergarten teacher pure hell. The mother was at her wits end and the tears flowed as she told me her story.

The teacher had indicated to the mother that she felt the problem was a lack of discipline in the home. This mother was a bright, well-educated woman, but in spite of all her education, she was no match for her little tornado. From the time he was a baby, her beautiful little son was in continuous motion. She said he has always "acted without thinking."

In my office, he crawled on the top of furniture, jumped from countertops, broke every toy in the playroom, and was, basically, uncontrollable. She had a leash she attached around his waist when they went out of the home, because he ran away from her. She could not keep him on a single task more than a minute or so. He was usually treated as a discipline problem, but punishment always made it worse. This type of pressure usually escalated the activity until he became uncontrollable and would physically lash out at the nearest person. Through her sobs, she said she was afraid that all of these problems were caused by her divorce and her status as a single mom.

Impulsivity, hyperactivity, and a poor attention span can be labeled Attention Deficit Hyperactive Disorder (ADHD). Even when I was able to get him to sit on the exam table, he was wiggling his foot. He was a beautiful little boy with sparkling

A Child is Waiting

eyes, black curly hair, a ready smile with deep dimples, and an inquisitive intelligence. When I examined him, he pulled on my stethoscope, turned the otoscope light on and off, searched my pockets, and was in constant motion. He could not control himself as his attention flipped from one thing to another.

Of course, all children who are overly active and have a short attention span and impulsivity do not have a specific syndrome called ADHD. The guidelines that have been established are: "the behaviors must be inconsistent with the child's age; they must appear before the age of seven and must be a problem in two or more areas in the child's life." Thomas met all of those criteria and needed help, now.

Various members of the school staff and the mother attended the Individual Education Plan (IEP) meeting at the school for Thomas, and a plan of management was developed. Everyone agreed that this problem was not due to his mother's divorce, not due to lack of discipline, and not due to excessive sugar intake, although these theories of dysfunction were discussed as maybe contributing to the problem.

The first report of children with these symptoms was written in Germany by Dr. Heinrich Hoffman in 1845. Dr. Hoffman was a poet, and he published a book titled *Slovenly Peter* or *Der Struwwelpeter.*

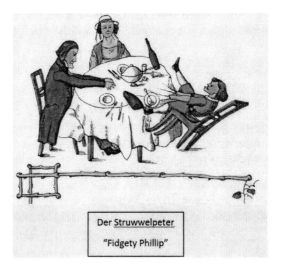

Der Struwwelpeter

"Fidgety Phillip"

In this book, he wrote a poem about his three-year-old son, "The Story of Fidgety Phillip." This poem captures the essence of attention problems better than anything written since. It was just like Thomas!

The IEP staff suggested a trial of medication. These children are often bright, and if the behaviors can be brought under control, they frequently excel in school. The mother agreed to a trial of medication and promised she would enroll in a support group and in a parenting skill training class.

The most effective medical treatment for decades has been the use of stimulant medication in combination with behavioral management. How the stimulant medication actually works in the brain has not been proven, but it is effective in many children. It has made it possible for some children with attention problems to adequately function in school and at home. The schoolteacher agreed to observe and to relate feedback regarding the effects of the medication. This is vital in order to regulate the dosage more effectively. With his excellent intelligence level, a supporting family, an understanding teacher, an effective medication, and quality communication between his teacher, his mother, and his doctor, he did extremely well.

Even though many children in my practice had problems in school, I must admit that this is not one of my special areas of knowledge. I will share a few of my ideas and leave you to your quest for knowledge to those who are much more experienced than me.

The concept that has been helpful in understanding learning difficulties in children has come to me from Melvin Levine, MD, a professor of pediatrics at the University of North Carolina and Director of the Clinical Center for the Study of Development and Learning. Maybe it will help you understand why a child may have trouble learning.

Each child is unique. No two are alike. Children are born with genetic inheritance from multiple past generations. The particular combination of DNA and genetic material in each child is influenced by the circumstances and environment into which he/she is born. There is no area that this is seen more clearly than the development of the nervous system, specifically the brain. This is called neurodevelopment and this development is critical to what, who, and why we are the individual that we are. The neurodevelopment starts with our genetic makeup but is altered, enhanced, or distorted by physical health, nutrition, social and cultural influences, emotional status, and other elements.

Each child is different, so it is no surprise that there is a wide variation in neurodevelopment. These variations are usually no problem because the majority of children find ways to handle the differences, although frequently help is required. When this variation becomes a weakness in acquiring a specific skill or learning a specific task, it becomes a dysfunction. A dysfunction that persists and blocks progress becomes a true disability. Untreated and continuing disabilities result in crippling handicaps. Most children can overcome a single dysfunction, but multiple dysfunctions usually will result in academic difficulties and require intervention.

When we consider neurodevelopment, it is helpful to recognize that we can analyze key elements in that developmental process. Dr. Levine lists eight areas that must be considered, including the strengths and weaknesses of each. Included in those eight are: memory, language, social cognition, neuromotor function, and attention. Of all of these, the one I have had the most experience with is attention. We are all aware of the diagnosis of ADD and ADHD. We continue to use these labels even though they are only descriptive of the symptoms that are interfering with the child's progress. They do not help us understand the underlying cause. However, when a distraught parent brings a child in with a specific dysfunction, that parent needs help and a search for answers must begin immediately.

Many dysfunctions in learning can add to the problem of attention difficulty. Only by addressing these specific areas can the problem of attention actually be corrected. For an example, a child with a language dysfunction may have semantic difficulty and trouble reading. That child certainly could have emotional stress, a short attention span, and could have trouble sitting still.

Only by correcting the language dysfunction will the attentional problem be helped.

From the age of five years, children spend a third of their lives in school. This represents a critical time in their developing personalities. It requires the intensive efforts of all who are in contact with them to see that the very best is accomplished. When the child's physician, who has been familiar with the child since birth, actively cooperates with the school in developing and implementing a program specifically designed to meet a child's individual needs, the child inevitably will benefit. The physician will have comprehension of the child's medical problems that may not be understood or known by the school personnel. Parents must encourage their child's doctor to participate in decisions affecting their child that are made by the school. At the same time, frequently, the school has information about the child that, when shared, helps the physician make appropriate and accurate medication treatments. In some conditions, such as autism, the families often desire more than the school can possibly give. The physician can help the school and the parents negotiate an understanding and a compromise, yet still find a path that will improve the child's functioning.

While we were trying to treat and conquer such diseases as meningitis, polio, measles, and other such dreaded illnesses, children who had trouble learning just were not a high medical priority. Most physicians have little knowledge of learning differences. Children who do poorly in school are often called lazy or poorly motivated. Blame is put on a "bad teacher" or a "poor school." More often, a parent is blamed for "lack of interest" or "not being involved." Occasionally, these statements are true, but for the many, there are serious problems in the child that prevent them from learning and progressing in school. In a society where education is directly related to success in the marketplace and the ability to earn a living, a learning dysfunction represents a crucial problem.

Attentional problems and many other dysfunctions do not just automatically disappear as we mature. In fact, if these dysfunctions are not addressed as children, they tend to get worse and certainly interfere with progress as we get older. They interfere with keeping a job, performance on a job, and many other areas critical to success in life.

Intervention starts with recognizing that there is a problem. A search for answers may lead to targeted help. It is important to take away the mystery of a lack of attention control. Help the child understand what is happening in their body. Use bypass strategy. Aim this at the specific point where the problem appears. For example, if the child has problems with numbers, find ways to help them use alternative methods to conquer the block. Counseling will help; especially, it will help the child understand the effects of the failures. Educational help, especially with testing, can often find a specific area of dysfunction that can be attacked. Last, medication can be used at any point, but it is not wise to wait until it seems there is no hope and then try medication as a last resort. By then, it is usually too late.

We must realize the disastrous results of learning dysfunctions that block the child from reaching their highest potential. These failures of intervention can doom an individual to struggles for the rest of their life.

CHAPTER TWENTY

Abuse and Neglect

The distraught young mother was holding her baby close to her chest. The infant was wearing only a diaper. He was having a seizure, the head pulled back, eyes turned to one side, and twitching movements all over the body. We worked feverishly for about twenty minutes to stop the seizure. After the seizure was controlled, the mother said the baby had been irritable all day and had recently gotten very quiet. She'd decided to come to our office, which was one block away from her home, when the baby started shaking. She said the baby was fine when she went to work and left it with the babysitter. The sitter had called her home when the baby vomited. The baby was very pale with a bluish cast to the skin. The soft spot on the head was open and swollen. The eye grounds revealed hemorrhages in the back of the eye. This was the case of the Shaken Baby syndrome, a tragic example of child abuse.

Someone had lost his or her temper and shaken the baby vigorously. This back and forth shaking causes a whiplash injury inside the brain and the blood vessels rupture, resulting in bleeding in the brain and in the eyes. The baby was admitted to the hospital and Child Protective Services and the police were notified. A *suspicion* of child abuse is enough to report to the local authorities. In fact, it is the law. Upon further examination, broken ribs and old bruises were found. This little innocent baby had been abused. The child lived, but the trauma resulted in brain damage, cerebral palsy, and blindness. He was damaged for the rest of his life.

How can a big, grown adult shake a tiny infant so violently that the blood vessels in the brain and eyes break and bleed? It happens. Daily, innocent children are subject to the anger and wrath of unthinking and uncaring adults. There is no punishment of the perpetrator that equals the suffering of that child. Besides, for the child, punishment of the perpetrator comes too late. The true answer is society must find ways to prevent such a crime from ever happening.

The challenges that face children all over the world are formidable blocks toward children achieving their rights. Physical abuse, emotional abuse, neglect, sexual abuse, poverty, hunger, lack of medical care, and diseases such as HIV/AIDS are among the most deadly.

A physical attack on the well-being of children often comes from those who should be protecting them. It is commonly perpetrated by a father, boyfriend, a baby sitter, or even the mother. Physical abuse, sexual abuse, and neglect are unforgivable. These attacks completely rob children of their rights and can ruin their lives. The damage is profound and usually will last throughout their lifetime. Certainly, if not physically, then emotionally.

The definition of neglect from *Safe Child* is clear:

> The neglected child is a child less than 18 years of age, who's mental, physical, or emotional condition has been impaired or is in danger of being impaired as a result of the child's legal guardian's failure to exercise a minimal degree of care in supplying the child with adequate food, clothing, shelter, education, or medical care. It also occurs when a child's legal guardian fails to provide the child with proper supervision or guardianship by allowing the child to be harmed or at risk to be harmed, which includes when the guardian uses drugs or alcohol him/herself.

The great psychiatrist Karl Menninger said, "What we do to children, they will do to society." The laws in every state of our union mandate that every citizen must report even the suspicion of neglect and abuse. The key word is ***suspicion***. When citizens become suspicious and do not report the situation to the proper authorities, they have broken the law, but more importantly, they have failed a child. Hundreds of thousands of children are abused, neglected, or damaged every day, and the resources to help them are woefully inadequate. In 2013, the American Academy of Pediatrics released a heartbreaking report that 3,188,000 cases of child abuse and neglect were investigated by Child Protective Services in the US Of those, 80 percent involve neglect, 18 percent involve physical abuse, 9 percent sexual abuse, and almost 9 percent were for mental abuse. One thousand five hundred and twenty of these children died. Yet, that may be only the tip of the iceberg, because many are not reported.

Perhaps the very best place to identify abuse is in the classroom. The classroom teacher knows her children better than any other person outside the home. This teacher can recognize when a child is suffering.

There are clear signs that indicate child abuse.
The child:

- Shows changes in behavior or school performance
- Has not received help for physical or medical problems
- Has learning or concentration problems not caused by a specific problem
- Is always watchful, waiting for something bad to happen
- Lacks adult supervision
- Is overly compliant, passive or withdrawn
- Comes to school early, stays late, and doesn't want to go home

The parent:

- Shows little concern for the child
- Denies there are problems, or blames the child for problems
- Asks teachers to use harsh punishment
- Sees the child as bad, worthless, or burdensome

- Demands an unreasonable level of academic or physical performance
- Looks to the child for care, attention, and satisfaction of their own emotional needs

These signs are not diagnostic but are signs that any person in the school or in the community of the child can easily see. They are definite indicators that a more in-depth evaluation is indicated. To act on signs without definite evidence is frightening, but each person must face their responsibility to the child.

Poverty is an insidious attack on our children and on families. The Coalition on Human Needs stated:

> In just one year the number of households in the United States that lacked the income for enough nutritious foods for their children rose from 36 million to 49 million including 17 million children. That is 4 million more in 2008 than in 2007.

This is an astonishing and overwhelming statistic. The greatest risk is in the very young and those who are fragile. The lack of nutrition leads to multiple problems, including the decreased ability to learn; problems in social, emotional, and behavioral interaction; poor physical health; and impairment in emotional development. The National Center for Children in Poverty has stated that, "Research is clear that poverty is the single greatest threat to the well-being of children."

Children do not make up a voting block in our society. They don't pay lobbyists or demonstrate in the streets. It is the responsibility of every citizen to lobby our government representatives including city, county, state, and federal agencies, to improve and increase the presently inadequate, overworked organizations that could possibly make a difference. Children should expect no less from those entrusted to protect them.

A video was released on YouTube showing a man, an elected judge, beating his teen-age daughter with a belt. It was obvious from the wild thrashing that he had lost control of his emotions and somehow thought he could beat his will, his opinion, or his idea of conforming into his daughter. It is difficult to understand how this could be called punishment or "a learning experience." If the adult does not show respect for a child, how is that child going to learn to show respect for others? Perhaps that is why an abused child often becomes an abuser parent.

In our society, the bickering politicians, the self-centered lobbyist, the opinionated journalist, and the disenfranchised public have left many of our children with inadequate nutrition, difficult to access health care, woefully inadequate health insurance, and a growing number of unprepared teen-age mothers. All of this, in a rich, highly educated nation. We, the public, can remedy some of these attacks on children by holding our politicians accountable at the ballot box.

The next time you have the opportunity to grade your congressman or -woman, evaluate whether they were active in protecting our children and vote carefully. That is called being a good parent, a concerned citizen, and a caring adult.

Sometimes it is difficult to "stick your neck out" even when the cause is right. This may be more than just reporting the suspicion of abuse. In the late 1970s, an opportunity to do more was presented to me and my wife, a psychologist.

The Child Protection Agency in Wichita, Kansas, asked us to evaluate cases of child abuse, neglect, and domestic violence. It would have been easy to plead "no time" or "I'm too busy," but those kids needed someone to be on their side. These cases were difficult, anxiety provoking, and full of emotion. Each one required a significant amount of time, but they were rewarding, especially if we could get the court to listen and act, or if various agencies were able to get the families to change. We spent hours in courtrooms, in depositions, with dysfunctional families, and with various agencies. Frequently, frustration was the emotion of the day, but never enough to make us quit, give up on a family, or abandon a court proceeding.

Testifying in court about an abusive relationship or about a neglected or abused child is anxiety provoking but a good way to reach a large number of people and articulate our view of the problems and the solutions. Frequently, reporters were there to inform the public of the proceedings. Sometimes while on the witness stand, I would see the abusive father or husband with hate-filled eyes glaring at me from his seat in the courtroom.

Once, there were two children, both little boys, brought in by a social worker for a physical evaluation. They had been beaten many times by their father while their mother watched. There were multiple severe injuries, including fractured bones, from past beatings. The father said to me, "This is none of your business. How I discipline my children is my business." He refused to admit it was wrong, was belligerent, and refused any suggestions of changes in behavior. The children were placed in protective custody, and we went to court. It was extremely difficult, but we recommended to the court that the children be removed from the home, the parental rights severed, and the children placed with the maternal grandmother. It was our opinion and that of others that this situation was hopeless.

The mother was crying and wringing her hands. The father glared at me and pointed his finger at me as if to shoot me. I felt fear, anxiety, and stress that caused tightness in my chest. Yet, I knew we were doing the right thing, as the children's welfare was the only thing that mattered. In this and in every case, we nourished the hope that the judge or the jury would be fair and just, with the welfare of the children always the presiding factor.

Occasionally, an opportunity to reach a large number of people happens and we must take an advantage of this chance to make a difference. This may be speaking out in a PTA meeting, writing a letter to the editor, helping a family in distress, or many other such adventures. It really doesn't matter whether you are helping one child, reporting a suspicion of abuse, volunteering to support children in the court system, mentoring a child after school, helping in a support group for parents, or writing a newspaper column. The need is great in all areas.

Being an advocate is merely being willing to step forward when the opportunity presents itself or even making your own opportunity.

CHAPTER TWENTY-ONE

Cancer

The word cancer brings out the worst fears that any parent can imagine. Actually, the word itself sounds awful. It's bad enough if it involves an adult, but when a child has the diagnoses, it just seems worse. Fortunately, many cancers of children have been, if not totally cured, at least brought under control. The wonderful research by children's cancer research centers around the world has resulted in miraculous results. Unfortunately, there are some that fall in the category of "We haven't found it yet."

For a bright little boy named Paul, this seemed to be true. Paul was twenty months old when he was first seen. He had lost weight, lost energy, was pale, and appeared ill. His abdomen looked swollen and was painful to the touch. His loving father carefully carried him and placed him on the exam table. A gentle palpation of his abdomen revealed a large mass. It was obvious we were dealing with a very serious condition. After talking with the parents about my fears, he was sent to the Children's Cancer Center, who confirmed the diagnoses of neuroblastoma. This is one of the bad guys of the children's cancer world.

Neuroblastoma is a cancer that develops from primitive embryonic nerve cells. It can occur anywhere in the body, but usually starts in the adrenal gland in the abdomen, creating a mass. As with most cancers, the cause is unknown. It is the third most common childhood cancer. These loving parents are now facing emotions only a parent who has suffered through a serious illness with their child can understand. Fear, guilt, blame, sadness, and anger flood into an entire family almost all at once.

A Child is Waiting

These are normal emotions but that doesn't make it any easier to face. The parents were told that Paul's cancer was in stage four, which meant it had spread beyond the primary tumor and was in his lymph nodes, bone, and bone marrow. In the majority of cases, this would represent an incurable cancer.

For Paul, there is a glimmer of hope, and this hope will carry him and his parents and his grandparents through some very difficult times. Chemotherapy and radiation therapy specially designed to kill the cancer cells will be started immediately. Stem cell rescue, utilizing his own bone marrow, hopefully will restore some of the normal cells after therapy. A new and exciting treatment has been developed that may give Paul a fighting chance. This treatment uses monoclonal antibodies to attack the cancer cells. These antibodies, called 3F8, are made by the white cells of mice. When given to a child, they attach to the cancer cells and the child's own immune system attacks the tumor. It's still in the research stage, but may improve Paul's chances if he can get it.

As we expected, Paul had reactions to the radiation therapy and lost weight. His little body was racked with nausea and vomiting. His energy level completely disappeared and he lost his hair. These attacks have not taken away his will to live and he is hanging on. Somehow, he manages to smile and even plays with his toy giraffe and teddy bear. His family members are amazing, spending every hour with him. His grandfather reads him story after story after story. The emotion that permeates that hospital room is hope. There are hundreds of cards pinned to the curtains around the room. There are visitors from uncles, cousins, and a Sunday school class, bringing small but welcome presents. More importantly, all bring a message of love and hope. Only time will reveal the final outcome.

Cancer in children is not rare. About one in 285 children will develop some form of cancer before the age of twenty. The American Cancer Society predicted 10,450 new cases and 1,350 deaths in children in 2014. They were extremely accurate. The most common cancers in children from 0 to fourteen are acute lymphocytic leukemia (26 percent), brain and central nervous system (21 percent), neuroblastoma (7 percent), and non-Hodgkin lymphoma (6 percent). The good news is that from 1975 the death rate has dropped over 50 percent. With the support of parents and a number of cancer related organizations, research in prevention and treatment is vigorous and ongoing. We look forward to the time that the 50 percent reaches 100 percent survival.

Acute lymphocytic leukemia (ALL) is the most common type of cancer in children.

When Mindy's teacher noticed that she couldn't keep with the other children in kindergarten, she mentioned it to the parents. They promised to help her get more sleep and rest. As time progressed, it got worse and she began to go to the school nurse with headaches and fever. Her physical exam revealed swollen lymph nodes in her axilla. The oncologist confirmed that it was acute lymphocytic leukemia.

The parents were devastated. They had hundreds of questions, many of them with no answers. The most important question was why did those white blood cells, called lymphocytes, suddenly start to multiply, choke off the bone marrow, and suck the life from this precious little girl. Unfortunately, we just don't know the answer to that question or any of the other "why" questions. But, even without the answers, there is hope.

This is a cancer of the bone marrow, the spongy center of the bones where all blood cells are made. The abnormal, immature white blood cells crowd out the normal disease-fighting white cells so that the body has problems fighting off infection. The red blood cells are also crowded out, so there are not enough to carry the oxygen necessary for life.

The word leukemia comes from the Greek *leukos* (white) and *haima* (blood). About one in a thousand children will develop ALL before the age of nineteen. Successful treatment consists of three phases of chemotherapy. The survival rate is now over 90 percent. It is crucial to include supportive care, monitor for infection, and maintain adequate nutrition.

Children undergoing therapy for cancer not only have the pain of the cancer itself but suffer from the fear and anxiety brought on by the treatment, hospitalization, separation anxiety, and psychological distress. Parents and other family members need help from the inevitable psychological distress. We must also never forget the pain, anxiety, and depression often seen in siblings as their brother or sister undergoes these frightening procedures.

As the chemotherapy killed off the cancerous cells, it also killed off some of Mindy's "good" cells. She was given a bone marrow transplant from a matched donor and it began to grow normal, non-cancerous cells. Mindy went into remission and began to act and feel like her usual self.

Mindy's parents signed on to one of the many cancer research center protocols. The results that were obtained for Mindy were added to the database of all cancer research centers and this helps oncologists continue to improve their choice of medications.

At this time, she is back in school and in remission. The parents realize that those cancer cells could start growing at any time, so they are ready to attack this monstrosity with all possible methods available. It is not completely successful in every case, but they are holding to the hope that Mindy will be in that 90 percent.

It is important for parents to recognize the early signs of cancer in their children. Early diagnosis can be a major factor in the results of therapy. St. Jude's Hospital has published the following list of warning signs that could be cancer or other serious illnesses.

- Fever
- Fatigue
- Listlessness
- Pallor
- Swellings or lumps
- Nausea or loss of appetite
- Insomnia or sleeping too much
- Whining or crying spells
- Stumbling or falling

- Double vision
- Frequent bruising
- Nosebleeds, or bleeding anywhere on the body

These are general symptoms and can be due to many causes. If they occur and are persistent, be sure that they can be explained. If they cannot, the child should be taken to the doctor to find the cause.

Conclusive scientific evidence documents that secondhand smoke is responsible for premature death and disease in children. The National Cancer Institute reports that children exposed to secondhand smoke are at risk not only for cancer but for Sudden Infant Death Syndrome (SIDS), acute respiratory infections, middle ear infections, severe asthma, and slowed lung growth. This is caused by a complex mixture of toxins in smoldering cigarettes and exhaled mainstream smoke. These toxins are formaldehyde, cyanide, carbon monoxide, ammonia, and nicotine. It has been shown that at least 250 chemicals in secondhand smoke are known to be toxic and/or cancer causing agents. The California Environmental Protection agency has reported that there are at least 430 SIDS deaths each year from secondhand smoke.

There is no such thing as a risk-free level of this smoke. Any level is dangerous. Cancer in children caused by this smoke is preventable by eliminating the smoke. It doesn't take a rocket scientist to understand this simple fact. The major exposures to children occur in the home or in the car. Intelligent adults who care for their children will stop this obvious attack on their children even if they choose to continue the attack on their own bodies. If you are one that may be causing an early death in your child, hear the child's plea and stop.

Note: The data and facts in this chapter were taken from the American Cancer Society Special Section: Cancer in Children and Adolescents.

CHAPTER TWENTY-TWO
Ethical Issues

The scientific and technical advances in medicine often outpace the ethical standards that society has accepted. In valiant attempts to guarantee children their right to good health, research has often taken us into uncharted territory. Frequently, this territory has created ethical and moral issues for individuals, organizations, and, in fact, all of society.

We saw that clearly when Dr. Fleming tried to convince the world that an extract from a simple mold could result in miraculous cures. He reported on the "bacterial killing quality of a mold called penicillin" in 1929. Society was not ready to accept that a mold could be useful and labeled him as a quack. It took ten years and the stimulus of a war to make his findings acceptable to everyone. Finally, in 1945, he was presented the Nobel Prize in Medicine for his discovery. It proved to be a miraculous cure. Not only did it provide a cure; it stimulated the development of over twenty classes of new antibiotics since penicillin became available.

Moral philosophy is the discipline concerned with what is morally good or evil or what is right or wrong. These terms are ambiguous and have different, conflicting interpretations in each individual, in each religion, and in each area of society. Abortion, genetic engineering, genetic population screening, stem cell treatment, and sometimes end-of-life care are some of the most controversial in our society today.

There is no greater example of this than what should happen in an unplanned, unwanted, undesired, accidental pregnancy.

The child was frightened, desperate, and kept her head down with eyes averted. She looked much younger than her fourteen years. Her mother was pacing around the room and looked at me with eyes, swollen with tears.

"What are we going to do? She's pregnant!"

I had been there when this child was born. She had been a month early and, as a preemie, had been in the neonatal unit for almost a month. Her parents called her their "miracle baby." We had been through many illnesses together. We had shared many wonderful experiences together. The school concert where she played a flute solo was delightful. Now that she is in middle school, I had not seen her as often. She was always a quiet child, a little shy and withdrawn. The whole family, including an older brother, attended church every Sunday and sometimes in between. The father was a banker and the mother a schoolteacher. The child was not promiscuous.

The entire family saw this as a tragedy and a devastating mistake that affected every member of the family. When she finally began to talk with me, she said, "I really don't know how it happened. We were just necking on the couch and it just happened. I know who the father is but I haven't told him. I'm scared. I'm so ashamed." Through her tears, she said she didn't want her boyfriend to know.

The mother said, "What can we do? Her life is over. Our lives are ruined. Our family is disgraced."

Unwanted, unplanned, undesired, or accidental pregnancies are a complicated and a difficult medical problem to manage. It is no longer a personal, individual, private event that can be managed between the family, the child, and their physician. It has become a major political, social, and religious conflict. Those who have never personally been faced with the problem, and even those who never will be personally faced with the problem, have developed strong opinions as to the "proper" or acceptable action to take.

Politicians use this medical event to gather votes. Ministers and priests discuss it as a sin or, sometimes, even to enrage their congregations. Television programs are written to increase ratings. It seems everyone would like to impose their own agenda and their own opinions on the unfortunate affected individual.

There are many facets to consider when faced with this dilemma. Perhaps the most difficult question to face is, when does this conception become a person or human life. At what point will the destruction of this pregnancy be labeled murder? Some believe it becomes a person at the moment the egg and sperm unite. Others believe it is after the cells divide and take on the shape of a fetus. Maybe it is when the heart begins to beat, or there is a reaction to pain. Could it be when the fetus could survive outside the mother's uterus? Some believe personhood begins when the infant is delivered and starts to breathe independently. There are even those who believe the egg or the sperm alone must be considered a person and with each menstrual period or each ejaculation, a baby is murdered. There are even those who believe that the use of contraceptives to prevent pregnancy is a sin. In actuality, there is no set definition or answer to any of these questions. There is no right or wrong. The answer lies in each person's opinion and the range is unlimited.

Unfortunately, the decision regarding the "proper" action is slowly eroding away from the pregnant individual, her family, and her medical consultant, and becoming a political football. It is even a major topic in our nation's presidential contest. It is important to remember that an unwanted and unplanned pregnancy usually results in an unwanted child. Unwanted children are frequently unloved, neglected, and abused. Should the abrupt, purposeful termination of the pregnancy at any stage be called murder? Should this pregnant teen be punished for getting pregnant or for having sex?

After calming this distraught family and finally helping them to think rationally, we began to look at their logical and legal choices. I told them that there are only three choices. Every choice has consequences that may not be acceptable, but never the less, one of these choices must be taken. She can have the baby and raise it with her parents, with or without the father's help. She can have the baby and give it up for adoption. She can terminate the pregnancy in a clean, sterile clinic. All three are legal and, though time is limited, there is still time for any one of these three choices. Any one of these choices is unacceptable to someone, some group, or some organization.

In the 1940s through the 1960s, before the "pill" and before sex education, many girls who became pregnant were forced by society and their families to live out their pregnancy in isolation in homes for unwed mothers. For many ostracized women, these homes were shame filled prisons. Adoptions were forced upon these unfortunate women. In the late 50s into the 60s, the process of adoption took a sinister turn. In 1964, a publication by the National Association of Social Workers stated "babies born out of wedlock are no longer a social problem . . . white, physically healthy babies are considered by many a social boon . . . [to adoption]." These women were treated almost as breeders.

Closed and forced adoptions were the norm. The mother rarely knew what happened to her baby after birth, creating long-term, delayed sadness, despair, and a sense of loss. Since that time, adoption has grown into a multi-million dollar business, virtually unregulated. In spite of this disturbing history, adoption is still a viable and positive alternative when managed with compassion and understanding. There are emotional and psychological consequences, but if managed correctly, these can be minimized.

Before the *Roe v. Wade* Supreme Court decision, many illegal back alley clinics, in the US and abroad, performed abortions, often with disastrous consequences. Young women were subjected to the possibility of infections, disfigurement, infertility, or death. As the pressure to halt "all" abortions mounts, legal and surgically acceptable clinics are becoming rare and difficult for the woman to access. The consequences may be the rise of illegal, back alley, unclean, and risky clinics, both in the US and beyond.

We recognize that an unwanted baby should not be brought into the world if it might be rejected, harmed, abused, neglected, or even killed. The answer must be found that is acceptable to the affected young woman and her family. It has been suggested that the "Plan B" pill may be the answer. This medication contains a female hormone that prevents ovulation and causes changes in the uterine lining, making it harder for the sperm to reach the ovum and for the fertilized egg to attach to the uterine wall. It is used to prevent pregnancy after unprotected sex or the failure of a birth control method. This pill must be taken within seventy-two hours of unprotected sex. It should not be used as a form of birth control. This is not the same as RU-486, which is a medication that induces abortions in the first trimester of pregnancy. Perhaps the prevention of pregnancy is the true answer.

When a pregnant teen receives counsel from her family, her physician, her spiritual advisor, or anyone else she decides to consult, does anyone, any legal authority, any religious body, or any individual have the right to force their personal beliefs on her? Should a woman be forced to go through pregnancy, labor, and delivery if it is not her choice? A pregnancy and delivery for a young teen is certainly a risky and potentially dangerous event for the mother and for the baby. Could it be that many in society believe that punishment for getting pregnant is indicated? Should the pregnant young woman be treated as a "bad" person? Some say she should be punished for having sex "out of wedlock."

Because of the conflicting range of opinions within each group of protesters and the cacophony that occurs around us, what is right for this unwanted, unplanned, and undesired pregnancy is lost. Meanwhile, the ego of the protesters, the self-image of the reporters, the economics of the media, the self-righteousness of the religious, and the self-aggrandizement of the politicos continue to fan the fires of discontent. This makes a viable and workable compromise within our society virtually impossible to reach.

Amid this confusion, the family, her doctor, and her religious counselor will help this young lady make the decision that is the best for her and her future, her family, and her pregnancy.

In another scientific dilemma, the advances in gene therapy have forced us to face the concept of right or wrong in the process of altering our basic genetic structure. Our genetic constitution is made up of those genes that have come to us from past generations. In a way, it is like having a piece of all your ancestors from all of your personal history. These genes actually tell our bodies who we are, what we look like, and what we are meant to be. We pass our genes, both healthy and flawed, down to our children, and they do the same to their children. It has been suggested that it is like immortality.

Scientists have now succeeded in mapping all the human chromosomes and many of those individual genes through the National Human Genome Project. We now have developed the expertise to alter many of those genes. This gene therapy has the potential to accomplish miracles in several ways. A normal gene can be inserted into a chromosome to replace a gene that has been determined to be abnormal, or an abnormal gene can be repaired through selective mutation. Genes can be turned on or turned off. This has already been done in cystic fibrosis and, if it is as successful as the reports indicate, this crippling disease of children could possibly be eliminated. Many other diseases, such as diabetes, heart disease, and cancer are being studied for possible gene therapy. Just as easily, science could utilize gene therapy to result in children being taller, or darker or lighter in skin pigment. Maybe the sex of your baby could be regulated. Possibly even sexual orientation. Would you like to order curly hair or straight hair; blonde, black, or red? Perhaps a dimple in the chin. We could call this designer babies.

The question for all individuals and for society is clear. How far should we go? What are the moral ethics of gene manipulation? Society could impose a collective will on the individual and dictate what is abnormal and what is normal. Should society have the power to tell the individual with cystic fibrosis that, even though we have the ability and the knowledge to alter the abnormal CF gene, society or government will not allow it, resulting in disastrous effects on that individual?

Through the human genome project every gene on every chromosome in the human body has now been discovered and plotted, although we still don't know the function of them all. This has the potential for unimaginable good for the human race. The challenge is to harness this power and information for progress.

We can genetically alter a potato to be resistant to the blight. Think what this could have done for Ireland in preventing the potato blight famine that killed thousands. We can genetically alter corn or wheat to be extremely more productive and feed millions of starving people. We can genetically alter cows to produce more milk. Do we have the right to impede the progress that has the potential to improve the human race, or does the fear of what "might" happen outweigh the good that "could" happen? Is it morally wrong to alter the basic building blocks of human kind even if they are flawed?

We are in the age of genomic medicine, and physicians and individuals now have the opportunity to participate in the new, personalized medicine. This is far removed from the past, when we searched for "cures" in the intense, crisis-driven treatment of "symptoms" medicine. We are rapidly approaching the reality of shifting medicine from the reactive to the predictive.

It is now possible to screen not only infants but entire populations for genetic information that will define the genetic possibilities in each individual. The implications of this are overwhelming. Soon we will be able to tell if an individual is susceptible to common problems such as diabetes, heart disease, or cancer. This has major implications as to who you should select as a mate, perhaps where you should live, or even what vocation you should choose.

Genetic population screening is not only possible but is actually being done. Tay Sacs disease is an inherited condition that only exists in Ashkenazi Jews. This is a severe, fatal, neurodegenerative condition that occurs when both parents are carriers of the abnormal gene. In 2000, it was reported that, worldwide, more than 1.4 million Jews have been tested and over 1400 couples have been identified to be at risk to have a child with this fatal disease. Many more have been identified since that time. With government intervention and intense reproductive counseling, pregnancies have been prevented or interrupted, and hundreds of affected infants have been avoided. Marriages have been prevented and even prohibited by the government.

Such population genetic population screening could possibly be done for diabetes, heart disease, cancer, and many other serious conditions. With this information, preventative measures could be undertaken before the condition even starts. Would this information be like a ticking bomb in the lives of each person? If a woman has the gene to develop breast cancer, should she have a perfectly normal, cancer-free breast removed to prevent what *might* happen? Many women have elected to choose this drastic measure.

Could issues of confidentiality be addressed effectively enough to protect the privacy of individuals? The 2008, Congress has passed a law to protect the privacy of the individual and to protect this information from being utilized against them. Unfortunately, this law will be difficult to enforce. This information could interfere with getting a job, influence who you choose to marry, block obtaining health or life insurance. It could result in disaster if the information were released. Lives could be ruined or drastically altered. Yet, lives could also be saved.

We must ask the question. Is it right to delve into the basic building blocks of all mankind? The potential for miraculous good is there, if society is ready. When we ponder the ethics of moral philosophy and the difference between good and evil or the difference between wrong and right, we must ask ourselves the basic question. In the field of medicine, is it right because we can? In the very near future, each of us may have the opportunity to make that decision.

There is no greater example of "if we can, should we" than in the world of stem cell research and treatment. This new and exciting treatment has tremendous possibilities in the future for correcting and treating many of the most serious illnesses and conditions affecting mankind. The possibilities of this momentous advancement became known to the general public when Christopher Reeves, our movie superman, suffered a catastrophic injury that severed his spinal cord. Researchers discussed the possibility of healing his spinal cord with stem cells.

In 1998, Dr. J.A. Thomson announced that he had isolated human stem cells from embryonic tissue. At the same time, Dr. J. Gearhart announced he had isolated human stem cells from fetal tissue. These announcements created the possibility of great medical breakthroughs. These stem cells have the possibility to be reprogramed into any tissue, organ, or type of cell. With a little imagination, the possibilities are endless. For example, it was suggested that these cells possibly could be implanted into Christopher Reeve's spinal cord to grow new cord cells and heal his cord. The therapeutic possibilities and promise of these cells after reprogramming for gene correction is exciting.

The origin of these cells alarmed many in all areas of society. Dr. Thompson's "human" cells came from embryos created in a fertility clinic. They were fertilized eggs that were going to be destroyed. They were five to seven days old and consisted of a mass of undifferentiated cells called blastocytes, or stem cells. Dr. Gerhardt's germ cell came from five- to nine-week old aborted fetuses. The ethical, political, and religious implications are enormous. It resulted in an attempt to stop all research in this field. For an individual with Parkinson's disease, multiple sclerosis, or Alzheimer's, the continuation of the research was critical and could be lifesaving.

There is no absolute answer that all will accept. The question remains. Is it right because we can? Do the results justify the means?

I will bring you another quandary to consider. In 2005, it was reported that a major break-through had occurred in the treatment of burns. When a child suffers second and third degree burns, it is necessary to graft skin onto the burned areas. Usually, the skin comes from the child and always results in scarring, contractures, and disfigurement. It is always very painful and requires multiple surgeries. In this new procedure, a small (3/4-inch) piece of skin is removed from a fourteen-week (about three inches long) aborted fetus and is grown to a much bigger size in the laboratory. This skin is then used for the graft. With fetal skin, there is no scarring, no contractures, and only minimal disfigurement. Healing is more rapid, and the child's suffering is reduced significantly. If the fetus is going to be aborted and destroyed anyway, is it right to use this tissue to benefit a burned child?

Maybe we should ask the burned child.

There are many more ethical quandaries to consider. The newest challenge has presented itself in the world of pharmacy. Many companies are conducting very expensive research, looking for cures. One company has developed a drug that will significantly improve the condition, extend the lifespan, and improve the lives of children with cystic fibrosis. This drug has now received the approval of the FDA. It will cost many thousands of dollars for a child to receive this miraculous treatment. The company must recoup its expenses in the development process, in the production, and in the distribution, and must realize a profit to stay in business. Can families afford to spend that amount of money? Can insurance companies pay an astounding amount of money? Should all taxpayers who fund the government pay for this treatment? This same process is happening in the treatment of cancer. We must find a way to settle this challenge because it is right to do so.

We have come a long way since my early days of holding the hand of a child with polio.

CHAPTER TWENTY-THREE

Parent Power

There has been much written about the power of parents. We have seen this power in the formation of numerous organizations dedicated to the improvement of their children's lives. Organizations founded by parents such as United Cerebral Palsy, The Muscular Dystrophy Association, Cure Autism Now, The Cystic Fibrosis Foundation, and many, many more have been influential in obtaining money for research, to support clinics and to influence governments. Sometimes, the goal was to obtain a specific program for their child, while other times it was to help thousands of vulnerable children.

In 1944, Tuleta, the daughter of John and Dela White, was born in San Antonio, Texas, with a profound congenital hearing loss. The Whites wanted her to learn to communicate by talking instead of using sign language. Dela White believed "if given the opportunity, children with hearing impairment could learn to listen, speak, and live a full, self-reliant life." However, there was no school in the area that taught hard-of-hearing children to use spoken language. It was the accepted method, at that time, to use only sign language. Even though she was a young mother, only twenty years old, Dela White had the love, willpower, and the foresight to search for and find a way to give these children the opportunity to remedy this deficiency in education.

She obtained financial and emotional support from local individuals and organizations and founded a school in San Antonio, Texas, whose primary goal was teaching hard-of-hearing children to listen and talk. When they painted a caretaker's cottage that had been donated as a schoolhouse with yellow paint, they named it the Sunshine Cottage. This school has grown significantly and has now become an internationally respected and accredited auditory/oral program for deaf and hard-of-hearing children. (Please see Chapter Thirteen.)

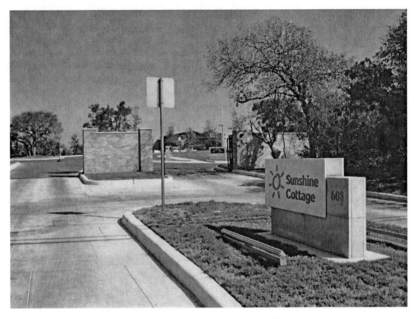

Entryway to Sunshine Cottage

For twenty-two years, Gordon Hartman developed his home building company into the largest home construction and land development company in San Antonio, Texas. In 2005, he sold his business and he and his wife established a foundation to pursue their dream of helping children and adults with special needs. Their daughter had been born with cognitive and physical needs.

In 2006, he noticed that even though his daughter wanted to participate in outdoor activities and play with other children, the facilities were always inadequate to encourage or even allow it to happen. His daughter was a pleasant, friendly child whose greatest desire was to see a smile on everyone's face. This desire became the inspiration for a father's dream to create "an oasis of friendship, a shrine of inclusion, an unforgettable wonderland for everyone," especially those with special needs and their families. The Hartman Foundation donated 15 million dollars and raised over 20 million dollars from interested contributors. In 2009, construction was started on Morgan's Wonderland, the first theme park in the world designed and constructed for the recreation and enjoyment of everyone, but especially for those individuals with special needs. At the grand opening, in April 2009, the park displayed twenty-five acres of rides, activities, and attractions. It is truly a wonderland built in the spirit of inclusion, where all ages and abilities can come together and have fun.

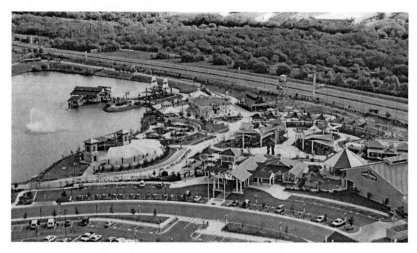

Aerial view of Morgan's Wonderland

The park now includes The Monarch Academy, a school for special needs children. To help support the park, Mr. Hartman has established a professional soccer team called The Scorpions. It is a member of the North American Soccer League, and when they play in their new stadium at the park, the proceeds help support the theme park. It is a unique but effective way to build lasting financial support. At their first home game, on April 15, over 17,000 people attended.

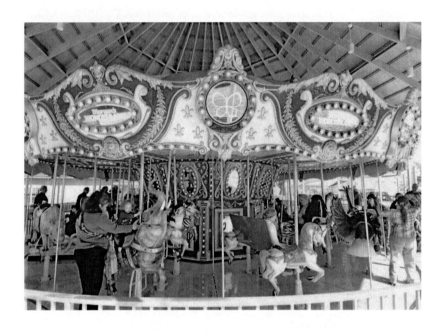

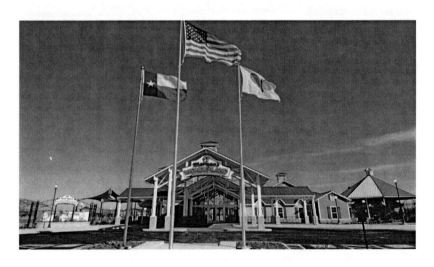

Entryway to Morgan's Wonderland

A Child is Waiting

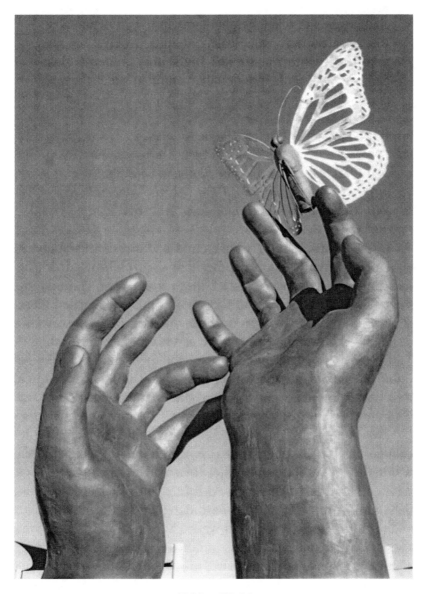

Taking Flight

Taking Flight dramatically symbolizes what Morgan's Wonderland stands for – to inspire those with special needs to soar beyond their physical or cognitive challenges and reach heights thought to be unattainable. Just as a butterfly magically emerges from a cocoon, unfurls its wings, and takes flight, this unique park is dedicated to each individual to dare to reach beyond their limitations and reach the heights of their dreams.

From the inscription on the plaque

A father's love for his daughter has made a significant contribution to all individuals, especially those with special needs and their families.

In the 1940s, parents whose child had a disability found it extremely difficult to obtain the help their child needed. The fear and misunderstandings of these vulnerable children by the medical community and the general public relegated these children to the level of second-class citizens. Many were institutionalized in warehouses and the parents told to "forget them." Those parents who decided to care for their children at home found a shocking absence of services and support. The children were not allowed to go to school and were isolated from the community. Families were isolated and felt alone and hopeless.

Two sets of parents came forward and made it possible to change the lives of thousands, even millions of these children and their parents. Jack and Ethel Hausman's son had been born with cerebral palsy. They joined forces with Leonard and Isabelle Goldenson, whose first-born daughter had cerebral palsy, and together they created what was to become a miracle for victims of cerebral palsy and their families for generations to come. The Goldensons and Hausmans had become millionaires from their hard work, and they put their ingenuity and work ethic into forming a new organization called The Cerebral Palsy Society. In 1948, they placed an ad in the *New York Herald Tribune* to recruit families interested in improving the services for their children. Hundreds of families joined with them to raise money to improve the care and the lives of these affected children. In 1949, the group became known as United Cerebral Palsy. UCP is probably the largest non-profit health organization in the United States.

The mission of UCP is "to advance the independence, productivity and full citizenship of people with disabilities through an affiliate network." Today, they have 100 service providers and reach more than 176,000 individuals and their families daily.

Those two sets of parents gathered more concerned parents and set into motion a program that has changed the lives of an untold number of children and adults.

Dr. Dan is an outstanding otolaryngologist (ear, nose, throat specialist). He has seen and helped thousands of children with cleft lip and cleft palate. His special talent is surgically repairing infants when they are born with this defect. Many are so severe that they cannot nurse and must be fed with an eyedropper. When his son was born without any defect, he cried with unrestrained joy. He was so grateful he thanked his God for the blessing. Then he started clinics across Mexico and Latin America to offer his surgical expertise to those unfortunate children who were born with a cleft palate. He said God had blessed him, so the least he could do was offer his talent to those children.

In 1920, a group of men who belonged to the Shriners division of Freemasons decided to start a new project to help children with disabilities. They established a group of non-profit hospitals to treat children with disabilities without charge to the family. The first hospital opened in 1922 in Shreveport, Louisiana. There are now twenty-two hospitals, including hospitals in Mexico City and Montreal, Canada. Three hospitals are dedicated to the treatment of children who have suffered burns. The staff consists of the highest quality of professionals available and many are on the staff of medical schools. Transportation to these hospitals is provided free of charge by Shriner-drivers across the country. Thousands and thousands of children have benefited from the expert care and treatment, at no cost, from these hospitals supported by these dedicated Shriners.

In 1950, the Scottish Rite of Freemasonry in Colorado initiated a program to help children with speech and language disorders. The overwhelming results of this program led to the establishment of RiteCare clinics throughout the United States. Today, there are 178 RiteCare clinics. As a rule, these clinics accept pre-school children who have difficulty speaking or understanding the spoken word or school-age children who have difficulty learning to read. These Scottish Rite men have stepped up and have improved the lives of many, many children.

It doesn't matter whether you are a member of a group, an individual with a child with a disability, or just a person who loves children. Any contribution you can make to improve the life of one child is the honorable thing to do. It takes the ability to recognize a problem and to be willing to do whatever it takes to help.

CHAPTER TWENTY-FOUR

Death

How dark the days seemed now, how sad and lonely the house and how heavy the hearts of the sisters as they worked and wait, while the shadow of death hovered over their once happy home! It was then that Margaret, sitting alone with tears dropping often on her work, felt how rich she had been in things more precious than any luxuries money can buy-in love, protection, peace and health, the real blessings of life.

From *Little Women* by Louise May Alcott, Chapter 18, "Dark Days"(Beth with Scarlet Fever)

Death is the inevitable outcome of life. A person will face death at some moment in life, whether it is a parent, a relative, a friend, a spouse, a child, or your own. Death brings out a myriad of emotions in those left behind, especially the caregivers. Feelings of sadness and loss are often mixed with the emotions of failure, inadequacy, guilt, and anger. Death reveals that there is a final step totally beyond our control. Many have problems facing this last step in life, even professionals who should be able to be more effective.

Celeste was a well-known professional, and a number of her friends and loved ones were gathered in the waiting room of the hospital. Her condition was critical and all who waited were anxiously waiting, hoping, and praying for good news. They all stood when the tall, distinguished physician entered the room. He was in a long, starched white coat that actually swished when he walked. Impeccably dressed, with a dark colored bow tie and a neatly trimmed moustache, he was the picture of professionalism.

"Well, she died. Any questions? If not, I have a lot to do."

They were stunned into silence as he turned and quickly left them standing in shock. Perhaps he felt anger that she had died, or maybe he felt guilt with his failure, or he may have had difficulty facing profound emotions. We don't know his feelings or his emotional status, but we do know that he was not in tune with those who deserved better.

When death happens, each survivor will react in their own unique way, and when it happens, it is the responsibility of each person to recognize and respect how the surviving loved ones respond. Some take comfort in their religion and it can be an uplifting experience. For others, it will be devastating and bring out pain or guilt or deep sorrow. Some will find strength in their family. Each individual must respect the responses of others as they integrate with their own personal feelings. It is important for each person to be in touch with their own responses to death because these feelings will be reflected in the attitude shown to the bereaving family.

The person who has done the most to help us understand our reactions to death and loss was Dr. Elizabeth Kubler-Ross. She was a psychiatrist and published her book, *On Death and Dying*, in 1969. Her research, her understanding, and her insight has brought many who were facing death to the stage of acceptance. Her quote that I love the most is as follows:

> You will not "get over" the loss of a loved one; you will learn to live with it. You will heal and you will rebuild yourself around the loss you have suffered. You will be whole again but you will never be the same. Nor should you be, nor would you want to be.

Death is not the only way to lose a loved one. Loss can happen due to a divorce, a stroke, a catastrophic illness such as dementia, or even a kidnapping or other such life altering experiences. The pain, grief, and heartbreak to such a loss can be just as difficult as a death.

Dr. Kubler-Ross has developed what she calls the stages of grief. These stages are a framework to help understand the reactions we experience after the loss of a loved one. Of course, each loss is different, just as each person is different, but these stages are a helpful start in coming to grips with the inevitable emotional turmoil we all feel. The stages she has described are denial, anger, bargaining, depression, and, finally, acceptance.

Denial is the first stage, and helps us survive the loss. In a prolonged illness, most individuals will face this stage before the death even occurs. It is quite normal to feel anger and to question "why." Some even feel that their god has deserted them. At this stage, we often blame someone or something that caused this death to occur. Following the denial, almost everyone will experience anger. This anger can extend to friends, doctors, hospitals, disease, oneself, one's god, or even the loved one who died. Anger has no limits, but we all are practiced in managing anger, so most of the time this anger will dissolve. Bargaining often occurs before the final event. Sometimes we bargain with god. "Please, god, if you will save this loved one, I will . . ." Probably the stage that is the hardest to recover from is the inevitable depression. Grief is part of depression and can last the longest of all the emotions we experience. Depression is a normal and necessary stage that we go through. It is a logical and realistic emotion to experience when a loved one is lost.

Each person will experience these stages for varying times and depths before the final acceptance. Acceptance is accepting the final reality that our loved one is really gone and will not return. This does not mean we like it or that things will be the same. We recognize that our lives have changed and we must go on living.

Each loss, each death, is different, and our reactions will be just as varied as the circumstances. A prolonged illness is certainly different from a sudden loss. As we move on in life, we must recognize that we are not betraying our loved one by learning to live without them being physically present. The memories will always be there, and we will cherish these memories as our loved one lives on in our heart and soul.

    In the saddest of circumstances, all we can truly offer is ourselves. We must acknowledge the feelings and emotions of those left behind, allow the expression of those emotions, and let them know that we are there with whatever support they can accept. Just be there for them and give of yourself.

Epilogue

The writing of these chapters has been a labor of love. As I remembered each child, I was filled with gratitude for being a part of their lives. I am grateful to those parents who gave me permission to include their stories. There were so many more that I wanted to include, but time and space made it impossible. This book has been written to bring the lives of children with developmental challenges to the forefront of every person's awareness.

It was not written for your enjoyment but to add to the understanding and knowledge that is vital to each individual, whether you are a parent, a therapist, a teacher, a family member, or just someone who loves children. However, I do hope you enjoyed it.

Here is my promise to children that has been my guide for over fifty years as a pediatrician.

I promise:

- That I will protect you from whatever or whoever tries to take away your right to happiness and joy.
- That I will care for you with the newest and most effective methods for any condition that interferes with your good health.
- That I will encourage and support you as you strive to reach your greatest potential.
- That I will guide your parents and extended family as they help you grow and develop through various stages of life.
- That I will listen to you, in whatever manner you choose to communicate with me.
- That I will be your friend, your supporter, and your helper as long as you desire.

Vernon L. James, MD

This book is the continuation of my promise to guide your parents, your caregivers, your therapist, your teachers, your doctors, and anyone else who also believes in the rights of children. These rights are: the right to happiness and joy, to safety and protection, to good health and effective treatment, and to the opportunity to reach their highest potential.

Vernon L. James, MD, FAAP

Index

A Quiet World P 79
Abortion P129
Abuse, physical/sexual/ emotional P116
Academic Achievement P77
Acceptance P147
Acute lymphoblastic Leukemia P123
Adaptive Behavior Scale P83
Adaptive communication P83
ADHD P110
Adoption P130
Adrenal Gland P122
Aids P56
ALS Foundation P70
American Eugenics Society P80
American Foundation of the Blind P105
American Print House for the Blind P105
American Society for Deaf Children P79
Angelman Syndrome P41
Angelman, Harry P41
Anger P147
Ashkenazi Jews P133
Asperger, Hans P88
Astigmatism P105
Asylums P105
Athetoid Dyskinesis P65
Audiology P73
Autism P86

Autism Diagnostic Interview P88
Autism Diagnostic Scale P88
Auto-immune condition P94
Autosomal Dominant Auto P74
Autosomal Recessive P74

Banting, Fred P96
Basal Metabolic Index P99
Behring, Emil Von P9
Best, Charles B P96
Bickel, Horst P24
Bilirubin P60
Bleuler, Eugene P87
Blind Harpist P105
Blindness P106
Botulism Toxin P65
Braille Alphabet P105
Braille, Louis P105
Brain Paralysis P63
Buck, Pearl P26-31
Burns P135

Calories P99
Canadian Organization for Rare Disorders (CORE) P28
Cancer P122
Case Western Reserve P89
CD 4 P57
Center for Autism and the Developing Brain P90
Cerebral Palsy P63
CFTR Gene P52

151

Children's Cancer Center P122
Civil Rights P82
Cleft Palate P143
Clinical Center for the Study of Development and Learning P112
Coalition on Human Needs P119
Cochlear Implants P77
Conductive Hearing Loss P76
Congenital Cataracts P107
Congenital Hearing Loss P75
Cowpox P16
CPK P67
Cranial Ultra Sonography P64
Cretin P28
Crocker, Allan P82
Crossed Eyes P104
Cure Autism Now P137
Cystic Fibrosis P50
Cystic Fibrosis Foundation P51
Cytomegalovirus (CMV) P59

Dahl, Roald P49
Deaf P73
Deafness P61
Death P145
Deletion, Gene P41
Denial P147
Denver Developmental ScreeningTest P28
Depression P147
Der Struwwelpeter P111
Designer Babies P132
Diabetes Mellitus P94
Diabetes Type I P94
Diabetes Type II P94
Diphtheria P8
Disability P113
Division of Handicapped Children P82

Down syndrome P32
Down, John Langdon P32
Drisapersen P70
Duchenne, Guillaune P68
Dysfunction P113
Dystrophin, Muscle Protein P70

Early Infant Development Program P42
Echolalia P87
Embryonic Nerve Cells P122
Enucleation P104
Erythroblastosis Fetalis P60
Eugenics P80

First World War P10
Folling, Asbjorne P23
Foster, Bryson P71
Fragile X P38
Freda, Vincent P62

Gallaudet University P82
Gene manipulation P133
Gene therapy P131
Genetic Population Screening P133
George Washington University P23
German measles P11
Gibson, William P108
Goldensen, Leonard P66
Gorman, John P62
Gowers Sign P67
Grief P147
Growth chart P99
Guthrie, Robert P27

Hand flapping P87
Handicap P113
Happy Puppet Children P41
Hard of hearing P79
Hartman, Gordan P138

Hausman, Jack P66
Hearing Aids P73
Hearing Loss P61
Hemolytic Disease of the Newborn P60
Herd Immunity P14
HIV P56
Hoffman, Heinrich P111
Holmes, Oliver Wendell P80
Holter valve P48
Holter, John P48
HRSA Global HIV/AIDS Program P58
Human Genome Project P132
Human life P129
Hydrocephalus P44
Hyperactive P110
Hyperglycemia P95
Hypoglycemia P95
Hypothyroidism P28
Hypertonia P65
Hypotonia P65

Impulsivity P110
Inbecellitis phenylpyruvica P23
Incubator, chick P19
Incubator, infant P19
Incubator, side show P19
Incurable P87
Individual Education Plan P111
Institute of Logopedics P64
Insulin P94
Intellectual Disability Disorder P80
Iron lung P1
Isolette P19-20

Jenner, Edward P16
Jerry Lewis P70
Johnson, Lyndon P82
Kalydeco P53

Kanner, Leo P88

Kaposi Sarcoma P57
Keller, Helen P106
Kennedy, John F. P82
Kernicterus P61
Ketoacidosis P95
Knights of the Blind P107
Koplik spots P15
Koplik, Henry P15

Language therapy P76
Lazy eye P107
Legal blindness P106
Levine, Mel P112
Lions Club International P107
Lord, Catherine P88
Lumacaftor P53

Macallister, Greg P11
Magnetoencephalography P89
Measles P14
Meconium Ileus P53
Medication Cost P136
Menninger, Karl P117
Meyers, David P79
Microcephaly P59
Middle/inner Ear P76
MMR P11
Monarch Academy P139
Mongoloid P32
Monoclonal Antibodies P123
Morgan's Wonderland P139
Mumps P10
Murder P129
Muscle biopsy P69
Muscular Dystrophy Association P69
Muscular dystrophy P67

New York Presbyterian Hospital
P88
National Center for Children in
Poverty P119
National Federation of the Blind
P105
National Foundation for Infantile
Paralysis P4
Neglect P117
Neonatologist P21
Neuroblastoma P122
Neurodevelopment P113
Neuro-developmental Disorder P87
Neuro-transmission P92
Newborn screening P75
NICU P20
Night writing P105
Nobel Prize 1923 P96
Non-Hodgkin Lymphoma P124

Obesity P99
Ophthalmology P104
Orchitis P10
Overweight P99

Pancreas P94
Parenting failure P101
Parotid gland P10
Personalized medicine P136
Personhood P129
Pertussis P14
Phenylketonuria/PKU P23
Phototherapy P61
Plague of Antoine P16
Plan B Pill P130
Pneumocystis caroni P58
Polio P2
Poverty P117
Prader-Willi Syndrome P43
Premature infants P18

Pseudohypertrophy P69
Public Law 85-126 P82
Public Law 88-164 P82
Public Law94-142 P82

Radiation therapy P123
Ramey, Craig P35
Recombinant DNA Insulin P96
Red measles P14
Red reflex P104
Retinoblastoma P104
Retinopathy of prematurity P106
Rh Factor P60
Rh Negative P60
Rh Positive P60
Right from Birth P35
RiteCare Clinics P143
Roe v. Wade P130
Roosevelt, Franklin D P4
Rotary International P5
RU 486 P131
Rubella P10
Rubeola P14

Sabin, Albert P4
Safe Child P117
Salk, Jonas P4
School for the Deaf P81
Scoliosis P45
Scorpion soccer P139
Scottish Rites P143
Seizures P116
Self-Help for Hard of Hearing
People P79
Self-injurious behaviors P87
Sensory hearing loss P74
Serapta Therapeutics P70
Shaken Baby syndrome P116
Shriners Hospitals P143
Shriver, Eunice Kennedy P84

Sight First P107
Silastic P48
Sleep apnea P100
Smallpox P15
Social cognition P113
Spastic diplegia P65
Spastic hemiplegia P65
Special Olympics P84
Speech Therapy P76
Spina bifida P44
Spitz, Eugene P48
Stem cells P123
Sterilization P81
Stimulant medication P112
Strabismus P107
Subsclerosing pan encephalitis P15
Sudden Infant Death (SIDS) P126
Sullivan, Anne P107
Sunshine Cottage P137
Suspicion of child abuse P116

Tay-Sacs Disease P133
Testicles P10
The Child Who Never Grew P31
The Good Earth P31
The Miracle Worker P107
The Story of My Life P107
The March of Dimes P4

Treacher-Collins Syndrome P74
Trisomy 13 P36
Trisomy 18 P36
Trisomy 21 P36
Tympanic membrane P76
Tympanometry P76

US Supreme Court P81
Ubiquitin P40
UNAIDS P58
United Cerebral Palsy P142
University of North Carolina P112
Unwanted child P127

Variolation P16
Vertex Pharmaceutical P53
Vineland social maturity scale P8
Visual impairment P61-106

Wardenberg syndrome P74
White, Dela P137
World Health Organization (WHO) P58
Whooping cough P13
Williams, William Carlos P8
World's Fair, Berlin P19

ZDV P57

Review Requested:
If you loved this book, would you please provide a review at Amazon.com?

CPSIA information can be obtained
at www.ICGtesting.com
Printed in the USA
FSOW01n0355030616
21099FS